Sports Anesthesia

Editor

ASHLEY M. SHILLING

CLINICS IN SPORTS MEDICINE

www.sportsmed.theclinics.com

Consulting Editor
MARK D. MILLER

April 2022 • Volume 41 • Number 2

ELSEVIER

1600 John F. Kennedy Boulevard ● Suite 1800 ● Philadelphia, Pennsylvania, 19103-2899

http://www.theclinics.com

CLINICS IN SPORTS MEDICINE Volume 41, Number 2
April 2022 ISSN 0278-5919, ISBN-13: 978-0-323-91994-4

Editor: Lauren Boyle
Developmental Editor: Diana Grace Ang

Clinics in Sports Medicine (ISSN 0278-5919) is published quarterly by Elsevier Inc., 360 Park Avenue South, New York, NY 10010-1710. Months of issue are January, April, July, and October. Business and Editorial Offices: 1600 John F. Kennedy Blvd., Ste. 1800, Philadelphia, PA 19103-2899. Customer Service Office: 3251 Riverport Lane, Maryland Heights, MO 63043. Periodicals postage paid at New York, NY and additional mailing offices. Subscription prices are $368.00 per year (US individuals), $959.00 per year (US institutions), $100.00 per year (US students), $409.00 per year (Canadian individuals), $988.00 per year (Canadian institutions), $100.00 (Canadian students), $480.00 per year (foreign individuals), $988.00 per year (foreign institutions), and $235.00 per year (foreign students). Foreign air speed delivery is included in all *Clinics* subscription prices. All prices are subject to change without notice. **POSTMASTER:** Send address changes to *Clinics in Sports Medicine*, Elsevier Health Sciences Division, Subscription Customer Service, 3251 Riverport Lane, Maryland Heights, MO 63043. Customer Service (orders, claims, online, change of address): Elsevier Health Sciences Division, Subscription Customer Service, 3251 Riverport Lane, Maryland Heights, MO 63043. **Tel: 1-800-654-2452 (U.S. and Canada); 314-447-8871 (outside U.S. and Canada). Fax: 314-447-8029. E-mail: journalscustomerservice-usa@elsevier.com (for print support); journalsonlinesupport-usa@elsevier.com (for online support).**

Reprints. For copies of 100 or more of articles in this publication, please contact the Commercial Reprints Department, Elsevier Inc., 360 Park Avenue South, New York, NY 10010-1710. Tel.: 212-633-3874; Fax: 212-633-3820; E-mail: reprints@elsevier.com.

Clinics in Sports Medicine is covered in *MEDLINE/PubMed (Index Medicus) Current Contents/Clinical Medicine, Excerpta Medica,* and *ISI/Biomed.*

Contributors

CONSULTING EDITOR

MARK D. MILLER, MD
S. Ward Casscells Professor, Department of Orthopaedic Surgery, University of Virginia, Charlottesville, Virginia, USA

EDITOR

ASHLEY M. SHILLING, MD
Associate Professor of Anesthesiology and Orthopedic Surgery, University of Virginia Health System, Charlottesville, Virginia, USA

AUTHORS

PETER E. AMATO, MD
Associate Professor, Medical Director, Acute Pain Service, Department of Anesthesiology, University of Virginia Health System, University of Virginia, Charlottesville, Virginia, USA

ALBERTO E. ARDON, MD, MPH
Department of Anesthesiology and Perioperative Medicine, Mayo Clinic, Jacksonville, Florida, USA

JAIME BARRATA, MD
Associate Professor of Anesthesiology, Department of Anesthesiology, Sidney Kimmel Medical College at Thomas Jefferson University, Philadelphia, Pennsylvania, USA

MELISSA CHAO, MD
Chronic Pain Fellow, Department of Anesthesiology and Pain Medicine, Columbia University Irving Medical Center, New York, New York, USA

BRITTANY DEILING, DO
Regional Anesthesia and Acute Pain Fellow, Department of Anesthesiology, University of Virginia Health System, Charlottesville, Virginia, USA

ANIS DIZDAREVIC, MD
Director of Regional and Orthopedic Anesthesia, Department of Anesthesiology and Pain Medicine, Columbia University Irving Medical Center, New York, New York, USA

BRETT ELMORE, MD
Assistant Professor, Department of Anesthesiology, University of Virginia Health, Charlottesville, Virginia, USA

GRACE L. FORSTER, BS
Department of Anesthesiology, Medical Student, University of Virginia Health System, University of Virginia, Charlottesville, Virginia, USA

RAJNISH K. GUPTA, MD
Vanderbilt University Medical Center, Department of Anesthesiology, Nashville, Tennessee, USA

NICOLE HOLLIS, MD
Assistant Professor, West Virginia University Department of Anesthesiology, Morgantown, West Virginia, USA

VIVIAN H. Y. IP, MBChB, MRCP, FRCA
Associate Clinical Professor, Staff Anesthesiologist, Department of Anesthesia and Pain Medicine, University of Alberta Hospital, Edmonton, Alberta, Canada

SIMRAT KAUR, DO
Anesthesia resident, Virginia Commonwealth University Medical Center Department of Anesthesiology, Richmond, Virginia, USA

JAMES KIM, MD
Assistant Professor, Department of Anesthesiology and Critical Care, Hospital of the University of Pennsylvania, Philadelphia, Pennsylvania, USA

PATRICK MEYER, MD
Assistant Professor, Department of Anesthesiology, University of Wisconsin, Madison, Wisconsin, USA

JEFFREY J. MOJICA, DO
Clinical Assistant Professor of Anesthesiology, Department of Anesthesiology, Sidney Kimmel Medical College at Thomas Jefferson University, Philadelphia, Pennsylvania, USA

CY MOZINGO, MD
Assistant Professor, West Virginia University Department of Anesthesiology, Morgantown, West Virginia, USA

KENNETH MULLEN, MD
Assistant Professor of Anesthesiology, Department of Anesthesiology, University of Virginia Health System, Charlottesville, Virginia, USA

GRANT NEELY, MD
Assistant Professor, West Virginia University Department of Anesthesiology, Morgantown, West Virginia, USA

AARON OCKER, DO
Clinical Instructor of Anesthesiology, Department of Anesthesiology, Sidney Kimmel Medical College at Thomas Jefferson University, Philadelphia, Pennsylvania, USA

MICHAEL O. ON'GELE, MD
Resident Physician, Department of Anesthesiology and Critical Care, Hospital of the University of Pennsylvania, Philadelphia, Pennsylvania, USA

CAROLE-ANNE POTVIN, MD, FRCPC
Clinical Assistant Professor, Staff Anesthesiologist, CHU de Québec – Enfant-Jésus and Saint-Sacrement, Quebec, Canada

VICTOR QI, MD
Resident Physician, Department of Anesthesiology and Critical Care, Hospital of the
University of Pennsylvania, Philadelphia, Pennsylvania, USA

ALESSANDRA RICCIO
Medical Student, University of Virginia School of Medicine, Charlottesville, Virginia,
USA

KAYLYN SACHSE, MD
Vanderbilt University Medical Center, Department of Anesthesiology, Nashville,
Tennessee, USA

KRISTOPHER SCHROEDER, MD
Professor, Department of Anesthesiology, University of Wisconsin, Madison, Wisconsin,
USA

ERIC S. SCHWENK, MD, FASA
Associate Professor of Anesthesiology and Orthopedic Surgery, Department of
Anesthesiology, Sidney Kimmel Medical College at Thomas Jefferson University,
Philadelphia, Pennsylvania, USA

DANIAL SHAMS, MD
Vanderbilt University Medical Center, Department of Anesthesiology, Nashville,
Tennessee, USA

CHRISTOPHER M. SHARROW, MD
Assistant Professor, Department of Anesthesiology, University of Virginia Health,
Charlottesville, Virginia, USA

ASHLEY M. SHILLING, MD
Associate Professor of Anesthesiology and Orthopedic Surgery, University of Virginia
Health System, Charlottesville, Virginia, USA

NICHOLAS STATZER, MD
Vanderbilt University Medical Center, Department of Anesthesiology, Nashville,
Tennessee, USA

BRYANT TRAN, MD
Regional and Acute Pain Fellowship Director, Virginia Commonwealth University Medical
Center Department of Anesthesiology, Richmond, Virginia, USA

MARISSA WEBER, MD
Clinical Instructor, Department of Anesthesiology, Weill Cornell Medicine, New York,
New York, USA

SARA WEINTRAUB, MD
Resident Physician, Department of Anesthesiology and Critical Care, Hospital of the
University of Pennsylvania, Philadelphia, Pennsylvania, USA

ANDREW J. WINKELMAN, BS
Department of Anesthesiology, Medical Student, University of Virginia Health System,
University of Virginia, Charlottesville, Virginia, USA

F. WINSTON GWATHMEY, Jr, MD
Associate Professor, Vice Chair for Education, Residency Program Director, Department of Orthopaedic Surgery, University of Virginia Health System, University of Virginia, Charlottesville, Virginia, USA

Contents

Athletes are among a unique group such that they may possess a serious underlying pathologic condition that may often go unnoticed given their high caliber of physical fitness. However, several considerations should be investigated, especially in the perioperative period, in order to minimize morbidity and mortality. Namely, cardiac pathologic condition can result in sudden death, and pulmonary pathologic condition may affect airway and respiratory management. Moreover, patients undergoing orthopedic surgery are at the highest risk for venous thromboembolism. Regardless of the condition, it is crucial to be vigilant and explore the unique medical considerations for the athlete undergoing anesthesia.

Upper extremity injuries are frequent in athletes which may require surgeries. Regional anesthesia for postoperative analgesia is important to aid recovery, and peripheral nerve blocks for surgical anesthesia enable surgeries to be performed without general anesthetics and their associated adverse effects. The relevant nerve block approaches to anesthetize the brachial plexus for elbow, wrist and hand surgeries are discussed in this article. There is very limited margin for error when performing nerve blocks and multimodal monitoring approach to reduce harm are outlined. Lastly, the importance of obtaining informed consent prior to nerve block procedures should not be overlooked.

Shoulder surgery introduces important anesthesia considerations. The interscalene nerve block is considered the gold standard regional anesthetic technique and can serve as the primary anesthetic or can be used for postoperative analgesia. Phrenic nerve blockade is a limitation of the interscalene block and various phrenic-sparing strategies and techniques have been described. Patient positioning is another important anesthetic consideration and can be associated with significant hemodynamic effects and position-related injuries.

Pain after hip arthroscopy can be severe, yet we lack a consensus method for non-narcotic analgesia. Here we describe anatomic elements of hip arthroscopy and our current understanding of the relevant sensory innervation as a prelude to the evaluation of locoregional analgesic techniques. Many regional nerve blocks and local anesthetic infiltration techniques are reviewed, including 2 newer ultrasound fascial plane blocks. Further study of targeted, motor-sparing approaches, either ultrasound-guided or under direct surgical visualization is needed.

Anesthesia for patients undergoing knee procedures encompasses a large patient population with significant variation in patient age, comorbidities, and type of surgery. In addition, these procedures are performed in vastly different surgical environments, including large academic hospitals, private hospitals, and out-patient surgical centers. These variabilities require a thoughtful and individualized anesthetic approach tailored toward the medical and surgical needs of each patient. This article discusses anesthetic approaches to patients with acute, subacute, and chronic knee-related pathology requiring surgery. We will also review pertinent knee anatomy and innervation and discuss regional nerve blocks and their applications to knee-related surgical procedures.

Modern anesthetic management for foot and ankle surgery includes a variety of anesthesia techniques including general anesthesia, neuraxial anesthesia, or MAC in combination with peripheral nerve blocks and/or multimodal analgesic agents. The choice of techniques should be tailored to the nature of the procedure, patient comorbidities, anesthesiologist skill level, intensity of anticipated postoperative pain, and surgeon preference.

Since 2018, the number of total joint arthroplasties (TJAs) performed on an outpatient basis has dramatically increased. Both surgeon and anesthesiologist should be aware of the implications for the safety of outpatient TJAs and potential patient risk factors that could alter this safety profile. Although smaller studies suggest that the risk of negative outcomes is equivalent when comparing outpatient and inpatient arthroplasty, larger database analyses suggest that, even when matched for comorbidities, patients undergoing outpatient arthroplasty may be at increased risk of surgical or medical complications. Appropriate patient selection is critical for the success of any outpatient arthroplasty program. Potential exclusion criteria for outpatient TJA may include age greater than 75 years, bleeding disorder, history of deep vein thrombosis, uncontrolled diabetes mellitus, and hypoalbuminemia, among others. Patient optimization before surgery is also warranted. The potential risks of same-day versus next-day discharge have yet to be elicited in a large-scale manner.

Patrick Meyer and Kristopher Schroeder

Elite athletes are exposed to an elevated risk of musculoskeletal injury which may present a significant threat to an athlete's livelihood. The perioperative anesthetic plan of care for these injuries in the general population often incorporates regional anesthesia procedures due to several benefits. However, some concern exists regarding the potential for regional anesthesia to adversely impact functional recovery in an elite athlete who may have a lower tolerance for this risk. This article aims to review the data behind this concern, discuss strategies to improve the safety of these procedures and explore the features of consent in this patient population.

Michael O. On'Gele, Sara Weintraub, Victor Qi, and James Kim

Local anesthetics have played a vital role in the multimodal analgesia approach to patient care by decreasing the use of perioperative opioids, enhancing patient satisfaction, decreasing the incidence of postoperative nausea and vomiting, decreasing the length of hospital stay, and reducing the risk of chronic postsurgical pain. The opioid-reduced anesthetic management for perioperative analgesia has been largely successful with the use of local anesthetics during procedures such as peripheral nerve blocks and neuraxial analgesia. It is important that practitioners who use local anesthetics are aware of the risk factors, presentation, and management of local anesthetic systemic toxicity (LAST).

Brittany Deiling, Kenneth Mullen, and Ashley M. Shilling

Continuous peripheral nerve block catheters are simple in concept: percutaneously inserting a catheter adjacent to a peripheral nerve. This procedure is followed by local anesthetic infusion via the catheter that can be titrated to effect for extended anesthesia or analgesia in the perioperative period. The reported benefits of peripheral nerve catheters used in the surgical population include improved pain scores, decreased narcotic use, decreased nausea/vomiting, decreased pruritus, decreased sedation, improved sleep, and improved patient satisfaction.

Danial Shams, Kaylyn Sachse, Nicholas Statzer, and Rajnish K. Gupta

Regional anesthesia has a strong role in minimizing post-operative pain, decreasing narcotic use and PONV, and, therefore, speeding discharge times. However, as with any procedure, regional anesthesia has both benefits and risks. It is important to identify the complications and contraindications related to regional anesthesia, which patient populations are at highest risk, and how to mitigate those risks to the greatest extent possible. Overall, significant complications secondary to regional anesthesia remain low. While a variety of different regional anesthesia techniques exist, complications tend to fall within 4 broad categories: block failure, bleeding/hematoma, neurological injury, and local anesthetic toxicity.

The success of enhanced recovery after surgery (ERAS) protocols in improving patient outcomes and reducing costs in general surgery are widely recognized. ERAS guidelines have now been developed in orthopedics with the following recommendations. Preoperatively, patients should be medically optimized with a focus on smoking cessation, education, and anxiety reduction. Intraoperatively, using multimodal and regional therapies like neuraxial anesthesia and peripheral nerve blocks facilitates same-day discharge. Postoperatively, early nutrition with appropriate thromboprophylaxis and early mobilization are essential. As the evidence of their improvement in patient outcomes and satisfaction continues, these pathways will prove invaluable in optimizing patient care in orthopedics.

CLINICS IN SPORTS MEDICINE

SERIES OF RELATED INTERESTED

Orthopedic Clinics
https://www.orthopedic.theclinics.com/
Foot and Ankle Clinics
https://www.foot.theclinics.com/
Hand Clinics
https://www.hand.theclinics.com/
Physical Medicine and Rehabilitation Clinics
https://www.pmr.theclinics.com/

THE CLINICS ARE AVAILABLE ONLINE!
Access your subscription at:
www.theclinics.com

Foreword

Anesthesia for Athletes

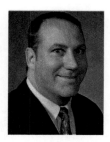

Mark D. Miller, MD
Consulting Editor

This issue of *Clinics in Sports Medicine* is not a pain, reaches well beyond a regional focus, and it won't put you to sleep! Although we often like to kid each other, Surgeons and Anesthesiologist are co-captains of the surgical team—we can't do our jobs without each other. Because athletes often present unique challenges to our anesthesia colleagues, I thought it was important to dedicate an issue of *Clinics in Sports Medicine* to this important topic. Therefore, I asked my "go-to" anesthesiologist (who I have also gone to for more than one surgery), Dr Ashley Shilling, to put together this issue that focuses on anesthesia for athletes.

This is a very thorough and well-organized treatise, beginning with introductory articles on special considerations for athletes and regional techniques and then progressing with a head-to-toe approach to anesthesia for each joint. It also includes well-written articles on local/regional anesthesia and, importantly, complications. The issue concludes with an article on multimodal analgesia, which we all need to promote in an effort to keep the opioid crisis off the field. Ashley and her team have done a phenomenal job with this issue. I would encourage every surgeon to get to know, and respect, their anesthesia team—all joking aside, they are an integral part of the team!

Mark D. Miller, MD
Division of Sports Medicine
Department of Orthopaedic Surgery
University of Virginia
400 Ray C. Hunt Drive
Suite 330
Charlottesville, VA 22908-0159, USA

E-mail address:
MDM3P@hscmail.mcc.virginia.edu

Clin Sports Med 41 (2022) xiii
https://doi.org/10.1016/j.csm.2022.01.001
0278-5919/22/© 2022 Published by Elsevier Inc.

Preface

Pulling Down the Surgical Drape Between the Anesthesiologist and the Orthopedic Surgeon...

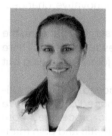

Ashley M. Shilling, MD
Editor

Since the first public demonstration of modern anesthesia in 1846, the field of anesthesiology has played a crucial role in all surgical specialties. The first spinal anesthetic (using cocaine) was performed in 1898 by August Bier, also the founder of the Bier block so frequently used in orthopedic surgery. Clearly, we have come a long way since cocaine spinals or even week-long admissions following anterior cruciate ligament surgery. Orthopedic anesthesia has evolved into an eloquent specialty that is efficient, safe, and evidence based. Modern-day orthopedic surgery may look something like this:

(1) A morning "breakfast" of Gatorade or black coffee
(2) Surgery in a state-of-the-art ambulatory surgical center complete with headphones, a personalized playlist, and possibly the avoidance of a general anesthetic
(3) Transitioning home from invasive surgery within only hours of surgery completion
(4) Recovery at home with a nerve block or continuous nerve catheter and multimodal analgesics
(5) Follow-up, including text messaging with the surgical and anesthesia providers, for postoperative care

In addition to modernizing perioperative care, another focus has been the integral and critical "team": the relationship between surgeon and anesthesiologist. Both parties must understand the procedure at hand and its related anesthetic options, including the potential for regional and neuraxial techniques and the risks of these and their alternatives. Both must appreciate patient comorbidities, the risks these comorbidities pose, as well as the surgical and anesthetic risks. Importantly, as more surgeries are shifting to outpatient settings, it is imperative that clinicians are creative and

Clin Sports Med 41 (2022) xv–xvi
https://doi.org/10.1016/j.csm.2022.01.002
0278-5919/22/© 2022 Published by Elsevier Inc.

sportsmed.theclinics.com

thoughtful with analgesic plans, including regional techniques, multimodal techniques, and ERAS (enhanced recovery after surgery) protocols.

At my institution, I am honored to be a part of a team collaboratively caring for orthopedic patients. Consistent care teams for orthopedic patients ensure optimal intraoperative care and perioperative outcomes. Studies indicate that medical teams decrease not only morbidity and mortality but also team burnout and medical errors. I like to believe that the invitation to contribute to the *Clinics in Sports Medicine* is an acknowledgment that we are all part of something not only collective but also vaster than our individual roles in patient care. I am fortunate to work with orthopedic surgeons who are not only talented but also welcoming, open to innovative changes, and fervent patient advocates.

While we have made incredible progress in the management of surgical patients, the field of anesthesiology continues to evolve, refining best practices for patients. There seems to be a new block technique emerging almost daily with journals pushing out new peer-reviewed studies faster than we can read them.

In the framework of these advancements, this journal is composed of several articles that pertain to the perioperative management of the orthopedic patient. We discuss anesthesia and pain management topics for orthopedic procedures from the shoulder down to the foot and ankle. We broach unique anesthetic and pain management considerations in caring for the elite athlete. We review modern joint arthroplasty, patient management in the ambulatory setting, and comprehensive perioperative care of the complex pain patient. Contributors from across the country have written articles specific to orthopedic anesthesia in hopes of fostering collaboration between fields and sharing relevant topics for the specialty of orthopedic sports medicine. Our hope is that this journal will offer something meaningful to every orthopedic surgeon.

No one can whistle a symphony. It takes a whole orchestra to play it.
— H.E. Luccock

Ashley M. Shilling, MD
Department of Anesthesiology
University of Virginia
PO Box 800710
Charlottesville, VA 22908, USA

E-mail address:
abm5f@hscmail.mcc.virginia.edu

Unique Medical Considerations for the Athlete Undergoing Anesthesia

Alessandra Riccio[a,1], Ashley M. Shilling, MD[b,*]

KEYWORDS

- Athlete • Anesthesia • Perioperative • Cardiac • Obstructive sleep apnea (OSA)
- Venous thromboembolism (VTE) • None per os

KEY POINTS

- It is not uncommon for athletes to have underlying medical conditions that may go unnoticed, proving to be devastating if not appropriately investigated.
- Several cardiac pathologic conditions unique to the athletic population often present asymptomatically and may cause sudden death without prodromal symptoms.
- Patients undergoing orthopedic surgery are at the highest risk for developing a venous thromboembolism.
- The main goal of the preoperative fasting guidelines set forth by the American Society of Anesthesiology Committee is to minimize the risk of perioperative pulmonary aspiration.
- A thorough history and physical examination, in addition to a keen foresight about the unique medical concerns surrounding athletes, are necessary to minimize morbidity and mortality in the perioperative period.

The connotation associated with the term *athlete* is often of a healthy individual who possesses physical agility, stamina, and strength. Although athletes are marked by their exceptional level of physical fitness, they often experience sports injuries that may require surgical intervention in which they will need to undergo anesthesia. This review highlights the unique medical concerns one should be aware of and investigate, specifically in the athletic population, in order to minimize morbidity and mortality in the perioperative period as the athlete undergoes anesthesia.

[a] University of Virginia School of Medicine, Charlottesville, VA, USA; [b] Department of Anesthesiology, University of Virginia Health System, MDPO Box 800710, Charlottesville VA 22908, USA
[1] Present address: 1 Rim Lane, Hicksville, NY 11801, USA
* Corresponding author.
E-mail address: 22908abm5f@virginia.edu

Clin Sports Med 41 (2022) 185–201
https://doi.org/10.1016/j.csm.2021.11.009
0278-5919/22/© 2021 Elsevier Inc. All rights reserved.

CARDIAC CONSIDERATIONS

Athletes are among a unique group in which normalcy may mimic disease. Because of this very concept, it is prudent to discuss cardiovascular adaptations associated with athletic training in order to highlight the disease states that should be considered and carefully evaluated in an athlete undergoing anesthesia. Namely, hypertrophic cardiomyopathy (HCM) and coronary artery anomalies, the 2 most common causes of sudden cardiac death (SCD) in athletes (**Table 1**), are highlighted.[1]

Physiologic Adaptations: Athletic Heart Syndrome

Athletic heart syndrome refers to the physiologic changes and cardiovascular adaptations associated with rigorous athletic training, specifically, ventricular dilation and bradycardia. First described in 1899 by the Swedish physician Henschen, cardiac enlargement was detected in Nordic cross-country skiers through auscultation and percussion. It was clear that athletes undergoing extreme combinations of endurance training experienced cardiac remodeling when compared with their sedentary counterparts.[2] In response to recurrent systemic oxygen deficits in the elite athlete, the left ventricular cavity increases in size in conjunction with hypertrophy of the left ventricle (LV) in order to maintain cardiac output. Importantly, left ventricular systolic function is usually normal. Manifestations of these structural adaptations can be detected by electrocardiogram (ECG), transthoracic echocardiography (TTE), and MRI, as seen in **Fig. 1**.[3] Any cardiovascular evaluation of an athlete must be performed with in-depth knowledge of the structural and functional cardiovascular changes associated with rigorous athletic performance, especially when attempting to diagnose specific cardiovascular conditions, such as HCM, discussed later, as there are many overlapping features between the natural physiologic state and a pathologic state (**Fig. 2**).[4]

Hypertrophic Cardiomyopathy

HCM, the leading cause of SCD in young athletes, is present in about 1 out of every 500 young adults (<35 years old).[5,6] It is crucial that this disease be at the forefront of diagnostic evaluation to achieve proper surveillance and treatment.

HCM, caused by an autosomal dominant mutation in one of the genes encoding the cardiac sarcomere, is characterized by a hypertrophied, nondilated LV with associated impairments in ventricular filling and compliance.[7] These structural abnormalities lead to asynchronized electrical impulses traveling throughout the myocardium

Table 1 Causes of sudden death in young athletes	
Cause	Percent
Hypertrophic cardiomyopathy	26.4
Commotio cordis	19.9
Coronary-artery anomalies	13.7
Left ventricular hypertrophy of indeterminate causation	7.5
Myocarditis	5.2
Rupture aortic aneurysm (Marfan syndrome)	3.1

Data from Minneapolis Heart Institute Foundation: Maron BJ, Shirani J, Poliac LC, Mathenge R, Roberts WC, Mueller FO. Sudden death in young competitive athletes: clinical, demographic, and pathological profiles. JAMA. 1996;276· 199-204.

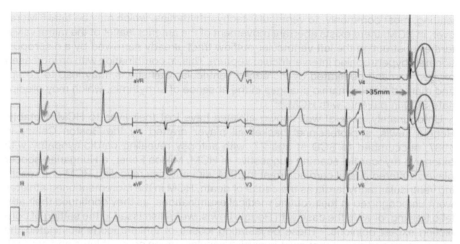

Fig. 1. The ECG of a 29-year-old male asymptomatic soccer player demonstrating sinus bradycardia (resting heart rate of 44 bpm). This ECG also demonstrates early repolarization in I, II, aVF V_2 to V_6 (*arrows*), voltage criterion for left ventricular hypertrophy (S-Vl + R-VS >35 mm), and tall, peaked T waves (*circles*). (Sharma S, Drezner JA, Baggish A, et al. International recommendations for electrocardiographic interpretation in athletes. Eur Heart J. 2018 Apr 21;39(16):1466–1480. doi:10.1093/eurheartj/ehw631. PMID: 28329355.)

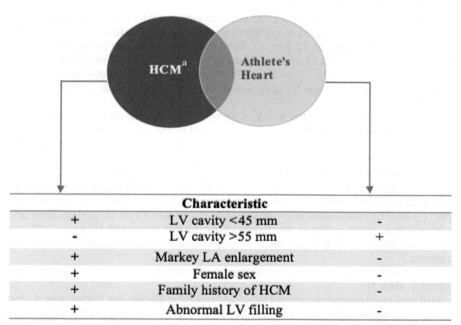

	Characteristic	
+	LV cavity <45 mm	-
-	LV cavity >55 mm	+
+	Markey LA enlargement	-
+	Female sex	-
+	Family history of HCM	-
+	Abnormal LV filling	-

Fig. 2. Differentiating HCM and physiologic cardiac changes in an elite athlete (athlete's heart). [a] HCM. (*Adapted from* Maron BJ. Distinguishing hypertrophic cardiomyopathy from athlete's heart: a clinical problem of increasing magnitude and significance. Heart. 2005;91 (11): 1380-13 82. doi: 10 .1136/hrt.2005. 060962)

leading, most commonly, to ventricular tachyarrhythmias, which may be fatal.[8] Moreover, in HCM, there exists aberrant movement of the anterior leaflet of the mitral valve, further obstructing the left ventricular outflow tract already narrowed by a disproportionately hypertrophied interventricular septum. This, in combination with an increased oxygen demand generated by increased ventricular wall stress, may lead to abrupt and marked hemodynamic changes in the absence of arrhythmia, which may precipitate SCD in patients with HCM.[5,9]

Unfortunately, several well-known athletes have lost their lives to HCM. Notably, Reggie Lewis, a professional basketball player drafted by the Boston Celtics in 1987, succumbed to SCD at age 27, with autopsy revealing cardiomyopathy with extensive myocardial scarring suggestive of HCM. Miklos Feher, a Hungarian soccer player, suffered a fatal cardiac arrest in 2004 with autopsy revealing HCM and resulting ventricular tachycardia as the cause of death. HCM in the aforementioned athletes went unrecognized in their routine medical examinations, as they continued their athletic training, or as in the case with Reggie Lewis, were dismissed in the setting of conflicting expert opinions.[7] These devastating losses of athletic icons illuminated the controversy and deficit that exist in cardiovascular screening in athletes and set forth the expectation of aggressive risk assessment.

For individuals with HCM, it is critical that medical clearance be obtained before participation in sports. Notably, only about 25% of competitive athletes who die suddenly have an underlying cardiac disease detected or suspected before participation in sports.[5] Thorough evaluation must begin with a personal and family history, as signs and symptoms may not be evident until teenage years. Although many patients with HCM may be asymptomatic, patients may present with symptoms related to left ventricular outflow tract obstruction, such as shortness of breath, chest pain, syncope, dizziness, palpitations, and unfortunately, SCD with most instances of sudden death clustering around peak times of competition. In a study of sudden death in 158 athletes between the ages of 12 and 40, 90% collapsed during or immediately after a training session with 36% of athletes meeting the criteria for HCM on postmortem autopsy. Furthermore, only 12 of the 158 athletes endorsed prodromal complaints further elucidating the need for appropriate evaluation in patients with HCM before athletic participation.[10]

Physical examination is also a crucial component, particularly in the evaluation of asymptomatic athletes with HCM, as a fourth heart sound may be the only abnormality to raise suspicion for an underlying congenital cardiac condition warranting further evaluation. It is important to note that physical examination may be normal in asymptomatic patients with occult HCM. Auscultation may also reveal a harsh crescendo-decrescendo systolic murmur beginning after S1, heard from the apex until the sternal notch along the left sternal border. This murmur may increase with a decrease in preload caused by maneuvers such as Valsalva and assuming an upright position after supine, sitting, or squatting as the degree of obstruction increases. However, although characteristic of HCM, this murmur may only be present in as few as 30% to 40% of patients.[11]

Clinical diagnosis of HCM is customarily made with 2-dimensional (2D) echocardiography (**Box 1**).

MRI may be of diagnostic value if echocardiographic studies are inadequate at identifying segmental hypertrophy.[12] Up to 75% of patients with HCM will have an abnormal ECG, even when echocardiography fails to demonstrate hypertrophy (**Box 2**).

Little evidence exists demonstrating a meaningful association between the ECG patterns of HCM and the left ventricular hypertrophy demonstrated on imaging.[11,13]

Box 1
Echocardiographic evidence of hypertrophic cardiomyopathy

- Hypertrophied but nondilated LV in the absence of other disease capable of producing that degree of hypertrophy

- LV wall thickness may range from mild (13–15 mm) to massive (>30 mm) (normal LV thickness ~ 12 mm)

Nevertheless, a combination of the aforementioned diagnostic studies should be used in the evaluation of patients with suspected HCM.

Although patient history and physical examination may provide the impetus for further diagnostic evaluation, there still exists many asymptomatic patients in which preparticipation screening for HCM remains a heavily debated subject for which there still does not exist a universally accepted paradigm. The 2020 American Heart Association (AHA)/American College of Cardiology (ACC) Guidelines for the Diagnosis and Treatment of Patients with Hypertrophic Cardiomyopathy recommends the following:

- Comprehensive cardiac history

- Family history, including 3 generations

- Comprehensive physical examination (including maneuvers such as Valsalva, squat-to-stand, passive leg raising, or walking)

The AHA/ACC recommends ECG and cardiac imaging only be pursued if clinical examination findings are highly suspicious of HCM.[14] However, an Italian study demonstrated a decrease in incidence of SCD between 1979 and 2004 in young competitive athletes (12–35 years old) since the introduction of a nationwide systematic screening, including a detailed patient and family history, physical examination, and ECG.[15] Clearly, there still is much room for discussion about the implementation of a more robust screening program in the United States.

Congenital Anomalous Coronary Artery

Congenital anomalous coronary artery is the second leading cause of SCD in athletes, accounting for 17% of young athlete deaths in the United States.[5,16] This congenital structural disease can be delineated into 2 types. The most common is the left main coronary artery arising from the right, or anterior, sinus of Valsalva, but there are instances whereby the right coronary arises from the left sinus.[5] A pivotal study conducted in 1974 documented that 27.3% of participants in whom the right and left coronaries arose from the anterior sinus experienced SCD. It was proposed that the acute leftward passage of the coronary artery along the aortic wall causes the entrance of the left coronary system to be slitlike (**Fig. 3**).[17] When the coronary sinus is subjected to aortic expansion, such as when there is increased cardiac output

---

Box 2
Electrocardiographic evidence of left ventricular hypertrophy

- ST segment and T-wave changes

- Large QRS complexes

- High-voltage R waves in the anterolateral leads (V4, V5, V6, I, and aVL)

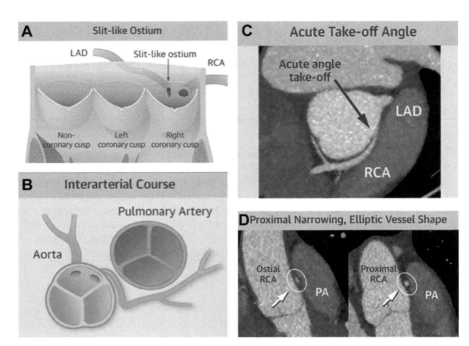

Fig. 3. (A) Slitlike orifice of the ostium of the coronary artery of the LAD versus the normal ostium of the RCA. (B) Course of the anomalous vessel between the aorta and pulmonary artery, allowing for entrapment and distal ischemia. (C) Acute take-off angle (<45°) of the proximal part of the coronary artery with a tangential course of the anomalous artery. (D) Proximal narrowing of the anomalous vessel with an elliptical shape. LAD, left anterior descending; RCA, right coronary artery. (*From* Grani C, Buechel RR, Kaufmann PA,Kwong RY. Multimodality Imaging in Individuals With Anomalous Coronary Arteries. JACC Cardiovasc Imaging. *2017;10(4):471-481*)

during exercise, the flaplike closure of the orifice stretches, leading to acute ischemia and fatal arrhythmia.[17,18]

One must be aware of this structural heart disease when evaluating athletes, as many are asymptomatic, and most will experience SCD either during or immediately after athletic exertion. A review completed in 2000 of 2 large registries of young, competitive athletes who died suddenly secondary to anomalous coronary arteries demonstrated that 55% of athletes had no clinical cardiovascular manifestations or testing during life. Those who did experience premonitory symptoms endorsed syncope and chest pain. All cardiovascular tests were within normal limits, including ECG, stress ECG with maximal exercise, and left ventricular wall motion and cardiac dimensions by 2D echocardiography.[19]

This raises the question of how to best diagnose a congenital anomalous coronary artery. It has been suggested that echocardiography would be the ideal simple, noninvasive, reliable method for detecting an anomalous origin of a coronary artery in asymptomatic athletes who do not warrant invasive testing.[20,21] Good interobserver reliability has been shown in observation of the coronary ostia and proximal course of the right and left coronary arteries with echocardiography. This suggests that coronary artery evaluation be included in any athlete undergoing a TTE for suspected cardiac disease, as imaging of coronary arteries is not routinely performed during standard adult TTE evaluations.[16] Importantly, the gold standard for diagnosing an anomalous coronary artery is computed tomographic (CT) angiography, which is a less suitable screening tool.[22] Once detected, it is recommended that the patient abstain from athletic training until appropriate risk stratification is pursued in determining the need for surgical correction.

PULMONARY CONSIDERATIONS

Although there appears to be a difference between exercise-induced bronchospasm (EIB) and exercise-induced asthma, the distinction is not always clear. Therefore, these terms are often used interchangeably. However, this review focuses on EIB, with a comparison to clinical asthma in the general population.

Exercise-Induced Bronchospasm

EIB, or the acute, transient airway narrowing occurring during exercise, occurs in 10% to 50% of athletes, particularly those involved in cold-weather sports.[23,24] Symptoms of EIB include chest tightness, shortness of breath, coughing, and wheezing, which may only be triggered by exercise without the typical features of asthma (nocturnal symptoms, frequent daytime exacerbations). This transient airway narrowing is a complex, multifactorial process that is primarily due to airway drying caused by a high exercise-ventilation rate. One hypothesis suggests that the inhaled dry air leads to water loss from the airway, causing a change in the airway lining osmolarity. This then leads to mast cell activation and subsequent secretion of inflammatory bronchoconstrictor mediators.[23] Another hypothesis suggests that bronchoconstrictor mediator release is caused by vascular engorgement as the airway rewarms after the inspiration of cold, low-humidity air during exercise.[24] This pathophysiology is thought to differ significantly from asthma seen in a clinic patient, as there is less allergic inflammation and therefore a weaker response to steroids in this disease state.

Athletes most at risk include those who compete in high-ventilation or endurance sports, such as cross-country skiing, swimming, and long-distance running. Moreover, environmental triggers, such as chlorine in pools and chemicals in ice rinks, may predispose athletes to developing EIB.[24] Aside from a comprehensive history to help distinguish EIB from other imitators, such as vocal cord dysfunction, allergic rhinitis, and cardiac pathologic condition, objective testing should also be pursued. Testing should begin with spirometry before and after bronchodilator therapy and will also help identify patients with concomitant asthma. However, many athletes with EIB will have normal baseline lung function, and spirometry may not reveal this underlying disease state. Therefore, bronchoprovocation testing is recommended (**Box 3**).

Pharmacologic and nonpharmacologic methods have been used in the treatment and prevention of EIB. Similar to asthma management, short-acting and long-acting β agonists, as well leukotriene modifiers, are useful pharmacologic therapies. The most common therapeutic recommendation to prevent symptoms of EIB is the prophylactic use of short-acting β agonists 15 minutes before exercise.[26] Ultimately, EIB often goes unrecognized and requires a keen diagnostician to properly investigate the signs and symptoms associated with EIB in order to prevent unnecessary respiratory distress in the elite athlete.

Given the high prevalence of underlying asthma in patients with EIB, it is important that asthma be optimally controlled before elective surgery. Although most anesthetics possess bronchodilating properties, patients with asthma are more prone to bronchospasm due to airway manipulation during intubation. Therefore, it may be

> **Box 3**
> **Techniques for diagnosing exercise-induced bronchospasm**
>
> - Eucapnic voluntary hyperventilation
>   - Decrease in forced expiratory volume in 1 second (FEV_1) of $\geq 10\%$ for positive result[25]
> - Hypertonic saline challenge
>   - Decrease in FEV_1 of 15% for positive result[25]
> - Methacholine challenge
> - Inhaled mannitol challenge test

beneficial to avoid general anesthesia and endotracheal intubation when possible. However, in instances where it is unavoidable, the use of a laryngeal mask airway has been shown to cause less airway reactivity than an endotracheal tube.[27]

Obstructive Sleep Apnea

Obstructive sleep apnea (OSA) is a chronic condition characterized by repeated upper-airway collapse during sleep, leading to nocturnal asphyxia and apnea, which in turn results in fragmented sleep, fluctuations in blood pressure, and increased sympathetic nervous system activity.[28] In both healthy persons and those with OSA, muscle tone of the genioglossus, the major dilatory muscle in the oropharynx responsible for maintenance of airway patency, is reduced at sleep onset. Therefore, individuals reliant on muscle tone in the setting of anatomic vulnerability are prone to obstruction of the upper airway during the transition from wakefulness to sleep. Hypoxia and hypercapnia ensue after collapse of the upper airway, resulting in an increase in sympathetic tone and subsequent patient arousal.[29] This cycle then occurs repeatedly throughout the night.

It is estimated that OSA occurs in 25% of women and up to 50% of men in the general population.[28] However, there is an alarming incidence of OSA within the athletic population that often goes unnoticed. In a study conducted on 257 retired National Football League players, sleep-disordered breathing was present in 52.3%, with a predominance in linemen.[30] Furthermore, another study demonstrated the prevalence of sleep-disordered breathing among all professional athletes to be 14% with a prevalence of 34% in linemen. Concordantly, linemen had the largest neck circumference and the highest body mass index (BMI).[31] These findings should heighten the clinical suspicion of OSA in athletes, as many have not considered such a diagnosis in young, healthy individuals who are in optimal physical condition.

The gold-standard diagnostic tool used in patients with suspected OSA is overnight polysomnography, which quantifies the number of apneas, defined by complete obstruction of airflow, and hypopneas, defined as a partial obstruction of airflow.[32] A detailed history marked by daytime sleepiness, snoring, witnessed apnea, poor concentration, headaches, moodiness, and irritability is suggestive of OSA. Risk factors for OSA include the following:

- Age greater than 40 years
- Male sex
- BMI greater than 35 kg/m^2
- Family history of OSA
- Hypertension
- Neck circumference greater than 16 inches

The semi-ubiquitous nature of these risk factors raises the question of whether to screen preoperative patients for OSA.

The guidelines and recommendations from the Society of Anesthesia and Sleep Medicine released in 2016 suggest a moderate level of evidence that OSA increases patients' risk for perioperative complications. Although there is little definitive evidence to support the benefits of preoperative screening, the expert recommendation for preoperative screening reflects the growing consensus in identifying patients at high risk for OSA before surgery in order to target perioperative interventions, which may help reduce patient complication. Therefore, the STOP-Bang questionnaire, a well-validated and extensively used screening tool, has emerged as one of the most commonly used screening questionnaires to help identify patients with OSA **(Fig. 4)**.[33,34] Other screening tests that have comparable accuracy include the Berlin questionnaire, the American Society of Anesthesiologists (ASA) checklist, and the-Perioperative Sleep Apnea Prediction Score (P-SAP) score.[35,36]

Importantly, OSA has been linked to many of the following postoperative complications:

- May result in intraoperative oxygen desaturation events and difficulty with intubation
- Development of atrial fibrillation
- Increased risk of cerebrovascular disease, such as stroke
- Development of pulmonary and systemic hypertension

With this, preoperative screening allows providers to use multimodal anesthetic and analgesic techniques, sparing benzodiazepines, narcotics, and general anesthesia whenever possible in order to avoid exacerbation of obstructive symptoms in the postoperative period.[35]

On a final note, the mainstay of treatment for OSA is the use of continuous positive airway pressure (CPAP), which provides continuous pressure during sleep to prevent upper-airway obstruction. Oral devices, such as mandibular advancement devices and tongue-retaining devices, are reasonable alternatives for patients who cannot tolerate CPAP. Numerous surgeries have also been proposed to correct obstructive anatomy, such as septoplasty, uvulopalatopharyngoplasty, epiglottoplasty, and maxillomandibular advancement.

STOP-Bang Questionnaire
Please answer the following questions by checking "yes" or "no" for each one

	Yes	No
Snoring (Do you snore loudly?)	☐	☐
Tiredness (Do you often feel tired, fatigued, or sleepy during the daytime?)	☐	☐
Observed Apnea (Has anyone observed that you stop breathing, or choke or gasp during your sleep?)	☐	☐
High Blood Pressure (Do you have or are you being treated for high blood pressure?)	☐	☐
BMI (Is your body mass index more than 35 kg per m^2?)	☐	☐
Age (Are you older than 50 years?)	☐	☐
Neck Circumference (Is your neck circumference greater than 40 cm [15.75 inches]?)	☐	☐
Gender (Are you male?)	☐	☐

Score 1 point for each positive response.
Scoring interpretation: 0 to 2 = low risk, 3 or 4 = intermediate risk, ≥5 = high risk.

Fig. 4. STOP-Bang questionnaire to assess the risk of OSA. (*Adapted from* Chung F, Abdullah HR, Liao P. STOP-Bang Questionnaire: A Practical Approach to Screen for Obstructive Sleep Apnea. Chest. 2016;149(3):631-638)

HEMATOLOGIC CONSIDERATIONS

Although preoperative laboratory testing is not universally indicated, specific laboratory studies are commonly ordered for preoperative evaluation, including a complete blood count (CBC), a basic metabolic panel, coagulation studies, and liver function studies. These tests may reveal an underlying anemia, thrombocytopenia, or coagulopathy that may warrant further diagnostic workup.

Disorders of Red Blood Cells

Anemia, marked by a reduction in the circulating number of red blood cells, is common among the US population. It is estimated that 3.5% of men and 7.6% of women in the United States are diagnosed with anemia, according to the most recent National Health and Nutrition Examination Surveys (2003–2012).[37] Those with mild anemia are typically asymptomatic; however, the threshold for experiencing sequelae of anemia is lowered in athletes, as their oxygen demand is higher, especially during performance. Symptoms of anemia include fatigue, shortness of breath, syncope, and generalized weakness. Therefore, it is important to identify the cause of anemia in order to reduce unnecessary hindrance on an athlete's activity.

The cause of anemia can be classified by either a decrease in production of red blood cells or an increase in destruction of red blood cells. The first diagnostic step in identifying the cause of anemia is obtaining a CBC. Once a low hemoglobin count is confirmed, the mean corpuscular volume (MCV) should be interpreted to classify the anemia as microcytic (MCV <80 fL), normocytic (MCV 80–100 fL), or macrocytic (MCV >100 fL).[38]

Microcytic anemias include iron deficiency anemia, anemia of chronic disease, and thalassemia. Iron deficiency anemia is by far the most common cause of anemia in the athlete, particularly among menstruating women. In addition to menstruation, iron deficiency may be secondary to gastrointestinal bleeding, hematuria, and sweating. Further workup for iron deficiency anemia includes serum iron, serum ferritin, total-iron binding capacity, and transferrin saturation, with a serum ferritin level less than 15 ng/mL highly suggestive of iron deficiency.[39] A study performed with Canadian endurance runners found that 29% of men and 82% of women had low ferritin levels (<25 ng/mL), although their hemoglobin and iron levels were normal.[40]

The diagnosis of thalassemia is confirmed via hemoglobin electrophoresis (β-thalassemia) or genetic testing (α-thalassemia).

- Workup for normocytic anemia includes calculating the corrected reticulocyte count to determine if there exists hemolysis or underproduction.

- Workup for macrocytic anemias includes a vitamin B12 and folate level as well as assessment for underlying liver disease.

This discussion would be incomplete without mention of mechanisms of anemia specific to athletes. One is dilutional pseudoanemia, which refers to a temporary increase in plasma volume during training that results in decreased hemoglobin concentration. Another involves intravascular hemolysis, termed "foot-strike hemoglobinuria," in which hemolysis is induced by the effects of contracting muscles on red blood cells.[41] Although athletes still remain susceptible to the aforementioned common causes of anemia, it is important to bear in mind unique mechanisms that exist in athletes.

Venous Thromboembolism

Thrombosis is the formation of a clot within a blood vessel, whereas an embolism is the migration of a clot. A common concern in postoperative patients is the development a deep venous thrombosis (DVT) and subsequent pulmonary embolism (PE) given the endothelial damage invoked on blood vessels during surgery and subsequent venous stasis during recovery, highlighting 2 of the 3 components of Virchow triad. Endothelial damage alters the dynamics of blood flow leading to turbulent flow within a vessel. Collagen is exposed, which triggers the extrinsic coagulation cascade, leading to platelet aggregation. Stasis, which results from postoperative pain or limb casting, allows the natural anticoagulant properties of blood to take effect as blood slows, leading to thrombus formation. The final component of Virchow triad is hypercoagulability. This inappropriate activation of the coagulation cascade may be inherited, such as with protein C deficiency, protein S deficiency, or hyperhomocysteinemia, or acquired, such as during pregnancy, while taking oral contraceptives, or in cancerous states.[42]

The physical exam for a DVT is quite unreliable with the classic findings of calf pain, warmth, and asymmetric leg swelling occurring in fewer than 50% of patients. Moreover, patients with a PE may be asymptomatic when less than 60% of the pulmonary circulation is obstructed, or may present with the classic signs of dyspnea, hypoxemia, and right heart failure in the setting of large occlusions. Therefore, a number of scoring systems have been devised to estimate the pretest probability of both a DVT and PE, with the most notable being the Wells Criteria (**Table 2**). [43,44,45,46] The clinical features of the Wells Criteria when assessing a DVT include:

- Active cancer (treatment or palliation within 6 months.
- Bedridden recently > 3 days or major surgery within 12 weeks.
- Calf swelling > 3 cm compared to the other leg (measure 10 cm below the tibial tuberosity).
- Collateral (nonvaricose) superficial veins present.
- Entire Leg swollen.
- Localized tenderness along deep venous system.
- Pitting edema, confined to symptomatic leg.
- Paralysis, paresis, or recent plaster immobilization of the lower extremity.[44,45,46]

Utilizing these criteria to stratify the clinical pretest probability into low, intermediate, or high, in addition to the clinical context, one can decide which of the various diagnostic modalities are best suited for the patient.

Patients undergoing orthopedic surgery are at the highest risk for developing a VTE. According to the American College of Chest Physicians, there is a 4.3% chance of VTE in the first 35 days after surgery in patients not receiving VTE prophylaxis, with the highest risk occurring in the first 14 days (2.80%).

Specifically, it is suggested that low-molecular-weight heparin (LMWH) be initiated 12 or more hours postoperatively and continued for 10 to 14 days, decreasing the VTE risk from 2.80% to 1.15%. Some literature supports the continuation of VTE prophylaxis for 35 days, decreasing the VTE risk to 0.65%. Of note, alternatives to LMWH include fondaparinux, low-dose unfractionated heparin, and adjusted-dose vitamin K agonists.[46] Although major orthopedic surgery increases the risk of VTE, most sports medicine procedures have minimal thromboembolic risk such that guidelines recommend against the use of routine chemoprophylaxis, and instead optimize early mobilization in patients who undergo joint arthroscopies and foot and ankle surgeries.[47–49]

Table 2
Wells score for deep venous thrombosis

Clinical Feature	Score
Active cancer (treatment or palliation within 6 mo)	1
Bedridden recently >3 d or major surgery within 12 wk	1
Calf swelling >3 cm compared with the other leg (measured 10 cm below tibial tuberosity)	1
Collateral (nonvaricose) superficial veins present	1
Entire leg swollen	1
Localized tenderness along deep venous system	1
Pitting edema, confined to symptomatic leg	1
Paralysis, paresis, or recent plaster immobilization of the lower extremity	1
Alternative diagnosis to DVT as likely or more likely	−2

Clinical pretest probability:
 Score total 0: Low
 Score total 1–2: Intermediate
 Score total ≥3: High
 Adapted from Wells PS, Anderson DR, Rodger M, et al. Evaluation ofD-dimer in the diagnosis of suspected deep-vein thrombosis. N WJld,..J Med. 2003;349(13): 1227-1235.

ENDOCRINE CONSIDERATIONS
Diabetes Mellitus

Athletes with diabetes mellitus (DM) may range from those participating in youth sports to those competing at the Olympic level, both of which present unique, yet difficult challenges to themselves and the health care providers managing their diabetes. Although 26.9 million people in the United States have been diagnosed with either type 1 or type 2 DM, exercising is often more complicated for those dependent on insulin, which encompasses all individuals with type 1 DM.[50] It is crucial that those caring for athletes with DM investigate the dietary patterns and the use of nutritional supplements and performance-enhancing drugs, as they may have detrimental effects on glucose management. For instance, insulin omission is a common practice in sports

Table 3
Wells score for pulmonary embolism

Clinical Feature	Score
Clinical signs and symptoms of DVT	3
Alternative diagnosis less likely	3
Heart rate >100 bpm	1.5
Previous PE or DVT	1.5
Immobilization at least 3 d or surgery in the previous 4 wk	1.5
Hemoptysis	1
Malignancy with treatment within 6 mo or palliative	1

Clinical pretest probability:
 Score total less than 2: Low
 Score total 2–6: Intermediate
 Score total ≥7: High
 Adapted from Wells PS, Anderson DR, Rodger M, et al. Evaluation of D-dimer in the diagnosis of suspected deep-vein thrombosis. *N Engl J Med.* 2003;349(13):1227-1235.

with weight categories, such as wrestling or boxing, in which athletes aim to lose weight before their weigh-in.[51] This undoubtedly results in poor glucose control and increases the risk of ketoacidosis.

Moreover, each type of exercise has its own effect on DM, with aerobic exercise resulting in hypoglycemia and bursts of anaerobic exercise leading to hyperglycemia. It is worthwhile to mention the phenomenon of delayed hypoglycemia, which occurs 6 to 12 hours after exercise with reports of cases presenting 28 hours after exercise. The pathophysiology involves depletion of glycogen stores after vigorous exercise followed by inadequate glycogen repletion, which, in the setting of a limited caloric intake in the postexercise interval, results in hypoglycemia as circulating blood glucose is extracted to replenish the depleted glycogen stores.[52] Several long-term complications also exist. They include microvascular complications, such as retinopathy, nephropathy, and peripheral neuropathy, as well as macrovascular complications, such as cardiovascular and cerebrovascular disease.

Diagnostic tests for diabetes mellitus include the following:

- Fasting plasma glucose levels
  - Less than 100 mg/dL: not concerning
  - 100 and 125 mg/dL: prediabetes
  - Greater than 200 mg/dL: DM
- Oral glucose tolerance testing
- Random plasma glucose levels

The main goal of treatment for DM centers on maintaining euglycemia and preventing hypoglycemia, which can cause significant morbidity and mortality in those with type 1 DM. Hypoglycemia should be treated immediately with the administration of glucose tablets or intravenous dextrose to prevent seizure and irreversible brain damage, as cerebral tissue is exceptionally metabolically active and thus heavily dependent on glucose. It is crucial for the athlete undergoing anesthesia to have appropriate glucose control, as hypoglycemia may be missed in patients who are anesthetized. Moreover, hyperglycemia contributes to poor wound healing and may result in an increased number of wound infections in the perioperative period.

NUTRITIONAL CONSIDERATIONS
None per Os Guidelines

The main goal of fasting in the preoperative period is to minimize the risk of perioperative pulmonary aspiration, which is defined as the aspiration of gastric contents occurring after the induction of anesthesia, during a procedure, or in the immediate postoperative period. The guidelines set forth by the American Society of Anesthesiology Committee on Standards and Practice Parameters in 2015 are limited to a healthy patient population undergoing elective procedures and do not apply to patients undergoing procedures without anesthesia or requiring only local anesthetics whereby upper-airway protective reflexes are not impaired, as they are not at risk for aspiration. The guidelines regarding the minimum fasting period described in **Table 4** are based on the gastric-emptying time of the ingested solids and/or liquids.[53] Enhancements in the quality and efficiency of anesthesia care continue to evolve to not only reduce the risk of aspiration but also decrease the risk of dehydration and hypoglycemia from prolonged fasting, minimizing perioperative morbidity.

Table 4	
American Society of Anesthesiologists fasting guidelines	
Liquid and Food Intake	**Minimum Fasting Period, h**
Clear liquids	2
Breast milk	4
Nonhuman milk	6
Light meal (toast, clear liquids)	6
Regular/heavy meal (fried/fatty food, meat)	8

Adapted from Practice Guidelines for Preoperative Fasting and the Use of Pharmacologic Agents to Reduce the Risk of Pulmonary Aspiration: Application to Healthy Patients Undergoing Elective Procedures: An Updated Report by the American Society of Anesthesiologists Task Force on Preoperative Fasting and the Use of Pharmacologic Agents to Reduce the Risk of Pulmonary Aspiration. *Anesthesiology.* 2017; 126:376–393.

SUMMARY

As outlined throughout this review, there are several unique medical considerations that exist for the athlete undergoing anesthesia. It is crucial to thoroughly review a patient's personal and family history as well as perform an in-depth physical examination, as many underlying conditions in the athlete may go unnoticed, which may increase the risk for perioperative mortality if the athlete were to undergo anesthesia.

DISCLOSURE

The authors of the current study certify that they have no affiliations with or involvement in any organization or entity with any financial interest (such as honoraria; educational grants; participation in speakers bureaus; membership, employment, consultancies, stock ownership, or other equity interest; and expert testimony or patent-licensing arrangements), or nonfinancial interest (such as personal or professional relationships, affiliations, knowledge, or beliefs) in the subject matter or materials discussed in this article.

REFERENCES

1. Maron BJ, Shirani J, Poliac LC, et al. Sudden death in young competitive athletes: clinical, demographic, and pathological profiles. JAMA 1996;276:199–204.
2. Thompson PD, Estes MNA. Ch 34: the athlete's heart. In: Topol EJ, editor. Textbook of cardiovascular medicine. 3rd edition. Lippincott Williams & Wilkins; 2007. p. 686–9.
3. Sharma S, Drezner JA, Baggish A, et al. International recommendations for electrocardiographic interpretation in athletes. Eur Heart J 2018;39(16):1466–80.
4. Maron BJ. Distinguishing hypertrophic cardiomyopathy from athlete's heart: a clinical problem of increasing magnitude and significance. Heart 2005;91(11): 1380–2.
5. Maron BJ, Epstein SE, Roberts WC. Causes of sudden death in the competitive athlete. J Am Coll Cardiol 1986;7:204–14.
6. Maron BJ, Gardin JM, Flack JM, et al. Prevalence of hypertrophic cardiomyopathy in a general population of young adults: echocardiographic analysis of 4111 subjects in the CARDIA study. Circulation 1995;92:785–9.

7. Bickel T, Gunasekaran P, Murtaza G, et al. Sudden cardiac death in famous athletes, lessons learned, heterogeneity in expert recommendations and pitfalls of contemporary screening strategies. J Atr Fibrillation 2019;12(4):2193.
8. Maron BJ, Adabag AS. Implications of arrhythmias and prevention of sudden death in hypertrophic cardiomyopathy. Ann Noninvasive Electrocardiol 2007;12:171–80.
9. Ross J, Braunwald E, Gault JH, et al. The mechanism of the intraventricular pressure gradient in idiopathic hypertrophic subaortic stenosis. Circulation 1966;34:558–78.
10. Maron B, Shirani J, Poliac LC, et al. Sudden death in young competitive athletes; clinical, demographic, and pathological profiles. JAMA 1996;276:199.
11. Kelly BS, Mattu A, William J, et al. Hypertrophic cardiomyopathy: electrocardiographic manifestations and other important considerations for the emergency physician. Am J Emerg Med 2007;25:72–9.
12. Maron BJ. Hypertrophic cardiomyopathy: a systematic review. JAMA 2002;287(10):1308–20.
13. Stroumpoulis KI, Pantazopoulos IN, Xanthos TT. Hypertrophic cardiomyopathy and sudden cardiac death. World J Cardiol 2010;2:289–98.
14. Ommen SR, Mital S, Burke MA, et al. 2020 AHA/ACC guideline for the diagnosis and treatment of patients with hypertrophic cardiomyopathy. Circulation 2020;142:558–631.
15. Corrado D, Basso C, Pavei A, et al. Trends in sudden cardiovascular death in young competitive athletes after implementation of a preparticipation screening program. JAMA 2006;296:1593–601.
16. Hoyt WJ, Dean PN, Schneider DS, et al. Coronary artery evaluation by screening echocardiogram in intercollegiate athletes. Med Sci Sports Exerc 2017;49:863–9.
17. Gräni C, Buechel RR, Kaufmann PA, et al. Multimodality imaging in individuals with anomalous coronary arteries. JACC Cardiovasc Imaging 2017;10(4):471–81.
18. Cheitlin MD, DeCastro CM, McAllister HA. Sudden death as a complication of anomalous left coronary origin from the anterior sinus of Valsalva. Circulation 1974;50:780–7.
19. Basso C, Maron BJ, Corrado D, et al. Clinical profile of congenital coronary artery anomalies with origin from the wrong aortic sinus leading to sudden death in young competitive athletes. J Am Coll Cardiol 2000;35:1493–501.
20. Pelliccia A, Spataro A, Maron BJ. Prospective echocardiographic screening for coronary artery anomalies in 1,360 elite competitive athletes. Am J Cardiol 1993;72:978–9.
21. Nakahara T, Takahashi-Tateno R, Hasegawa A, et al. Doppler echocardiography may provide a potentially life-saving screening of anomalous origin of coronary artery in young athletes. Int J Cardiol 2012;156:104–5.
22. Hauser M. Congenital anomalies of the coronary arteries. Heart 2005;91:1240–5.
23. Rundell KW, Jenkinson D. Exercise-induced bronchospasm in the elite athletes. Sports Med 2002;32:583–600.
24. Holzer K, Brukner P. Screening of athletes for exercise-induced bronchoconstriction. Clin J Sport Med 2004;14:134–8.
25. Molis MA, Molis WE. Exercise-induced bronchospasm. Sports Health 2010;2:311–7.
26. Sinha T, David AK. Recognition and management of exercise-induced bronchospasm. Am Fam Physician 2003;67:769.
27. Brimacombe J. The advantage of the LMA over the tracheal tube or facemask: a meta-analysis. Can J Anaesth 1995;42:1017–23.

28. Chung F, Heinzer R, Vat S, et al. Prevalence of sleep-disordered breathing in the general population: the HypnoLaus study. Lancet Respir Med 2015;3:310–8.

29. Eckert DJ, Malhotra A. Pathophysiology of adult obstructive sleep apnea. Proc Am Thorac Soc 2008;5:144–53.

30. Albuquerque F, Sert Kuniyoshi F, Calvin A, et al. Sleep-disordered breathing, hypertension and obesity in retired National Football League players. J Am Coll Cardiol 2010;56:1432–3.

31. George C, Kab V, Levy A. Increased prevalence of sleep-disordered breathing among professional football players. N Engl J Med 2003;348:367–8.

32. Semelka M, Wilson J, Floyd R. Diagnosis and treatment of obstructive sleep apnea in adults. Am Fam Physician 2016;94:355–60.

33. Chung F, Yegneswaran B, Liao P, et al. STOP questionnaire: a tool to screen patients for obstructive sleep apnea. Anesthesiology 2012;108:768–75.

34. Chung F, Abdullah HR, Liao P. STOP-bang questionnaire: a practical approach to screen for obstructive sleep apnea. Chest 2016;149(3):631–8.

35. Chung F, Memtsoudis SG, Ramachandran SK, et al. Society of Anesthesia and sleep medicine guidelines on preoperative screening and assessment of adult patients with obstructive sleep apnea. Anesth Analg 2016;123:452–73.

36. Ramachandran SK, Kheterpal S, Consens F, et al. Derivation and validation of a simple perioperative sleep apnea prediction score. Anesth Analg 2010;110:1007–15.

37. Le CH. The prevalence of anemia and moderate-severe anemia in the us population (NHANES 2003-2012). PLoS One 2016;11:e0166635.

38. Maner BS, Moosavi L. Mean corpuscular volume. In: StatPearls. Treasure Island, FL: StatPearls Publishing; 2020.

39. Guyatt GH, Oxman AD, Ali M, et al. Laboratory diagnosis of iron-deficiency anemia: an overview. J Gen Intern Med 1992;7:145–53.

40. Clement DB, Asmundson RC, Medhurst CW. Haemoglobin values: comparative survey of the 1976 Canadian Olympic team. Can Med Assoc J 1977;117:614–6.

41. Selby GB, Eichner ER. Endurance swimming, intravascular hemolysis, anemia, and iron depletion. New perspective on athlete's anemia. Am J Med 1986;81:791–4.

42. Kushner A, West WP, Pillarisetty LS. Virchow triad. In: StatPearls. Treasure Island, FL: StatPearls Publishing; 2020.

43. Stone J, Hangge P, Albadawi H, et al. Deep vein thrombosis: pathogenesis, diagnosis, and medical management. Cardiovasc Diagn Ther 2017;7:S276–84.

44. Siegal D, Lim W. Ch 142: Venous thromboembolism. In: Hoffman R, editor. Hematology: basic Principles and practice. Elsevier; 2005. p. 2102–12.

45. Wells PS, Anderson DR, Rodger M, et al. Evaluation of D-dimer in the diagnosis of suspected deep-vein thrombosis. N Engl J Med 2003;349(13):1227–35.

46. Falck-Ytter Y, Francis CW, Johanson NA, et al. Prevention of VTE in orthopedic surgery patients: antithrombotic therapy and prevention of thrombosis, 9th ed: American College of Chest Physicians Evidence-Based Clinical Practice Guidelines. Chest 2012;141(2 Suppl):e278S–325S.

47. Iahi OA, Reddy J, Ahmad I. Deep venous thrombosis after knee arthroscopy: a meta-analysis. Arthroscopy 2005;21:727–30.

48. Jameson SS, Augustine A, James P, et al. Venous thromboembolic events following foot and anklesurgery in the English National Health Service. J Bone Joint Surg Br 2011 Apr;93(4):490–7. https://doi.org/10.1302/0301-620X.93B4.25731. PMID: 21464488.

49. Geerts WH, Pineo GF, Heit JA, et al. Prevention of venous thromboembolism: the seventh ACCP conference on antithrombotic and thrombolytic therapy. Chest 2004 Sep;126(3 Suppl):338S–400S. https://doi.org/10.1378/chest.126.3_suppl. 338S. PMID: 15383478.
50. National diabetes statistics report, 2020. Atlanta, GA: Centers for Disease Control and Prevention, U.S. Dept of Health and Human Services; 2020.
51. Harris GD, White R. Diabetes in the competitive athlete. Curr Sports Med Rep 2012;11(6):309–15.
52. MacDonald MJ. Postexercise late-onset hypoglycemia in insulin-dependent diabetic patients. Diabetes Care 1987;10:584–8.
53. Practice guidelines for preoperative fasting and the use of pharmacologic agents to reduce the risk of pulmonary aspiration: application to healthy patients undergoing elective procedures: an updated report by the American Society of Anesthesiologists Task Force on preoperative fasting and the use of pharmacologic agents to reduce the risk of pulmonary aspiration. Anesthesiology 2017;126: 376–93.

Regional Anesthesia for Athletes Undergoing Upper Extremity Procedures
Techniques and Considerations

Carole-Anne Potvin, MD, FRCPC[a],
Vivian H.Y. Ip, MBChB, MRCP, FRCA[b],*

KEYWORDS

- Regional anesthesia for upper extremity
- Different approaches to brachial plexus block • Nerve blocks in athletes
- Multimodal monitoring approach

KEY POINTS

- Upper extremity injuries are common, and almost half of these injuries are fractures. Different techniques are available to anesthetize the brachial plexus for these upper extremity surgeries.
- Regional anesthesia offers analgesic benefits, early mobilization, improved rehabilitation and patient satisfaction. Open discussion to obtain informed consent and reiterate risks before nerve block procedure is essential.
- Multimodal monitoring approach should be used to minimize intraneural injection during nerve block performance since there is very limited margin for error.
- In the presence of coagulopathy or bleeding diathesis, performing brachial plexus blocks where the nerve is in close proximity to noncompressible arteries is NOT recommended.
- Rebound pain should be recognized and managed with multimodal transitional pain pathways and patient education in the pre-operative setting.

INTRODUCTION

Upper extremity injuries represent 35% of sports-related injury, and close to 45% of these injuries are fractures.[1] Hand and wrist injuries are particularly common, and

^a CHU de Québec – Enfant- Jésus & Saint-Sacrement, 1050 Ch Ste-Foy, Québec, QC, G1S 4L8, Canada; ^b Department of Anesthesia and Pain Medicine, University of Alberta Hospital, 2-150 Clinical Sciences Building, Edmonton, Alberta T6G 2G3, Canada
* Corresponding author.
E-mail address: hip@ualberta.ca

Clin Sports Med 41 (2022) 203–217
https://doi.org/10.1016/j.csm.2021.11.003
0278-5919/22/© 2021 Elsevier Inc. All rights reserved.

prompt treatment is often required to increase the chances of full functional recovery.[1,2] Acute elbow injuries (fractures, dislocations) are mostly seen in contact sports, and chronic injuries tend to be overuse in nature. The treatment of most elbow injuries will be conservative; however, some will require surgeries for fracture and instability reduction.[3] Athletes can also present with stress fractures, albeit relatively rare compared with lower extremities. For the upper extremity, ulnar fracture is the most frequent bony injury.[4]

As the athletes prepare for surgery, the risks and benefits of each procedure should be considered so patients can make an informed choice of the most suitable type of anesthesia and analgesia specific to their operation. Regional anesthesia may allow patients to avoid the need for general anesthesia (GA) and its associated side effects and can help improve pain management and facilitate a faster recovery.[5] However, regional anesthetic techniques can be associated with the risk of nerve injury, a catastrophic outcome that can affect both the career and livelihood of athletes. Therefore, it is essential for athletes to have an uncoerced, open discussion about the risks and benefits of each anesthesia technique with their regional-trained anesthesiologist in order to formulate an individualized management plan.

PERIPHERAL NERVE BLOCKS FOR UPPER EXTREMITY SURGERY

Analgesia for surgeries below the clavicle can be provided by supraclavicular, infraclavicular, or axillary blocks.[6,7] The choice between the different approach will be influenced by surgical site and patient-related factors including body habitus and sonoanatomy. Different dermatomes will be covered by each technique, as demonstrated in **Fig. 1**.

DIFFERENT TYPES OF ULTRASOUND-GUIDED NERVE BLOCKS FOR UPPER EXTREMITY SURGERIES

For elbow, wrist, and hand surgeries, the brachial plexus can be blocked at multiple locations as outlined.

Supraclavicular Nerve Block

For the supraclavicular nerve block (SCB), the patient is positioned supine with the head turned toward the contralateral side and the ipsilateral arm stretched down by the side of the body. A high-frequency linear transducer (15–6 MHz) is placed in the supraclavicular fossa to obtain a short-axis view of the subclavian artery. The divisions (and sometimes trunks) of the brachial plexus can be observed typically on the posterolateral side of the artery. It is important to visualize the first rib *lateral and deep* to the artery and nerve bundle (**Fig. 2**) and to take note of the pleura to avoid inadvertent pleural puncture, as the needle is advanced lateral to the artery. Using a 22G insulated nerve block needle in an in-plane technique, with a lateral to medial approach, local anesthetics (LA) (20-25mL in total) will be injected at the junction between the first rib and the nerves, and then in between each section of the nerve bundle.[7] To minimize multiple needle injection, which may potentially increase risk of needle trauma to the nerve bundle, 2 injections are recommended: one at the 7 o'clock position to the artery and the other at 10 o'clock position to the artery (see **Fig. 2**).

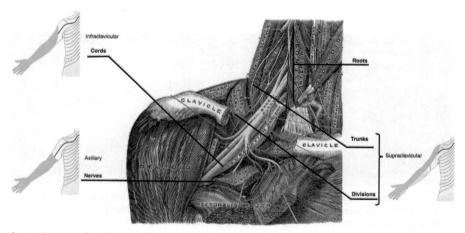

Fig. 1. Sensory distribution for the supraclavicular, infraclavicular, and axillary nerve blocks.

Supraclavicular Nerve Block	
Advantages	**Disadvantages**
Easily identifiable sonoanatomy.	Easy to miss the ulnar distribution.
Can produce quick and effective surgical anesthesia.	Potentially difficult in obese patients, as the structures are deep and the pleura is in close proximity to the block needle target.
	Aberrant vessels such as suprascapular artery or the transverse cervical artery can be in close proximity or along the path of the needle.

Tips and pearls—supraclavicular nerve block
• Position the first rib deep to the subclavian artery and the brachial plexus on the lateral side.
• Use hydrodissection to increase space between the divisions and highly recommend using multimodal monitoring approach (outline later) to prevent intraneural injection.
• Tilting the transducer can aid image optimization.

Infraclavicular Nerve Block

For the infraclavicular nerve block (ICB), the patient is positioned supine with the head turned toward the contralateral side. The ipsilateral arm can be stretched down by the side of the body or abducted with the elbow flexed at 90° to accentuate the cords of

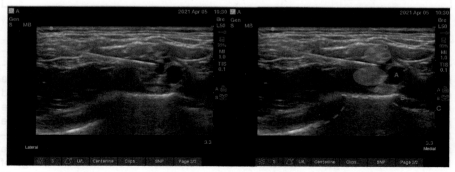

Fig. 2. Ultrasound image showing the sonoanatomy of the supraclavicular nerve block. (A) Supraclavicular artery; (B) first rib; (C) pleura; (D) trunks/divisions of the brachial plexus; (E) nerve block needle.

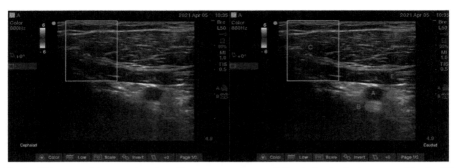

Fig. 3. Ultrasound image showing the sonoanatomy of the infraclavicular nerve block. (A) Axillary artery; (B) lateral, posterior, and medial cords of the brachial plexus; (C) thoracoacromial artery; (D) pectoralis major muscle; (E) pectoralis minor muscle.

the brachial plexus by raising the clavicle and reducing the depth of the nerves. A high-frequency linear transducer (15–6 MHz) is placed sagittal, inferior to the coracoid process in the infraclavicular area to obtain a short-axis view of the axillary artery. In this approach, the structures are deep and can be found under the pectoralis major and pectoralis minor muscles. If the pleura is visualized, the transducer may be too medial; therefore, it can be positioned or simply tilted laterally where the axillary artery and the surrounding cords can be visualized without the pleura deep to them. Most of the time the lateral, posterior, and medial cords of the brachial plexus can be visualized at 9 o'clock, 6 o'clock, and 3 o'clock from cephalad to caudad, respectively, surrounding the axillary artery (**Fig. 3**). It is important to identify the thoracoacromial vessel (using the color Doppler) between the pectoralis muscles, potentially in the needle trajectory (see **Fig. 3**). LA (25-30mL) will be injected just posterior to the axillary artery above the posterior cord, and the operator will look for the double-bubble sign[6] or a U-shaped distribution of the LA around the artery.[7]

Infraclavicular Nerve Block	
Advantages	**Disadvantages**
Preferable location for nerve block catheter insertion because the pectoralis muscles aid "anchoring" the nerve block catheter in situ.	Deep block with the coracoid process making needle manipulation challenging.
Tips and pearls—infraclavicular nerve block	
• Note the thoracoacromial artery within the needle path.	

Costoclavicular Nerve Block

The costoclavicular nerve block is a relatively new alternative approach to the infraclavicular block. The patient is positioned supine with the head turned toward the contralateral side. The ipsilateral arm is abducted and elbow flexed 90° to accentuate the cords of the brachial plexus. A high-frequency linear transducer (15–6 MHz) is placed transversely or transverse-obliquely *immediately* caudad to the clavicle to visualize the axillary vessels between the clavicle and second rib. At this level, the cords of the brachial plexus are clustered lateral to the axillary artery (**Fig. 4**). The block is performed by advancing the needle from a lateral to medial direction and injecting the LA (25-30mL) in the gap between the lateral and posterior cord.[8] The advantage of this block, compared with the ICB, is that all the cords are close together at a relatively superficial location with the serratus anterior muscle underneath the plexus as a

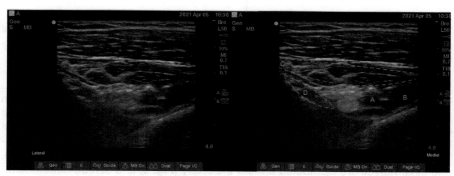

Fig. 4. Ultrasound image of the sonoanatomy of the costoclavicular nerve block. (A) Axillary artery; (B) axillary vein; (C) subclavius muscle; (D) serratus anterior muscle. (L) Lateral, (P) posterior, and (M) medial cords of the brachial plexus.

"safety cushion." The disadvantage is the potential lack of space for needle maneuver due to the proximity of the transducer to the coracoid process. Furthermore, this area can be vascular, especially if the transducer is positioned further caudad to the clavicle. The cephalic vein, axillary vein, and other branches of the axillary artery, for example, the superior thoracic artery or the thoracoacromial artery can be visualized.

Costoclavicular Nerve Block	
Advantages	**Disadvantages**
Preferable location for nerve block catheter insertion because the pectoralis muscles aid "anchoring" the nerve block catheter in situ. Relatively easy block with single injection in between all the cords, as they are in close proximity.	Similar to infraclavicular block, the coracoid process can make needle maneuver challenging; therefore, medial to lateral approach can be considered.
Tips and pearls—costoclavicular nerve block	
• Note the aberrant vessels in close proximity.	

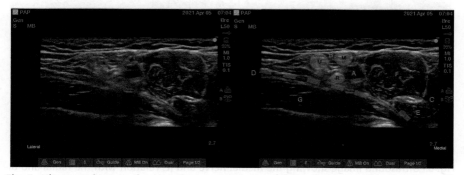

Fig. 5. Ultrasound image showing the sonoanatomy of the axillary nerve block at the axilla apex. (A) Axillary artery; (B) median, ulnar, and radial nerves; (C) musculocutaneous nerve in the coracobrachialis muscle; (D) conjoint tendon; (E) coracobrachialis muscle; (F) biceps muscle; (G) latissimus dorsi muscle; (M) median nerve; (U) ulnar nerve; (R) radial nerve.

Note of caution for supraclavicular, costoclavicular, and infraclavicular blocks
The arteries referenced in supraclavicular, infraclavicular, and costoclavicular brachial plexus blocks are noncompressible; therefore, they are not recommended to be performed on patients with coagulopathy or bleeding diathesis.[9]

Axillary Approach to Brachial Plexus Nerve Block

For the axillary brachial plexus block (AXB), patients are placed supine with the arm abducted at 90°. A high-frequency linear transducer (15–6 MHz) is placed at the *apex* of the axilla to obtain a short-axis view of the axillary artery at the level of the conjoint tendon of the latissimus dorsi and teres major muscle. The musculocutaneous nerve is situated inside the coracobrachialis muscle. The radial, median, and ulnar nerves are distributed around the artery (**Fig. 5**) and can be better identified by scanning the arm from proximal to distal to "trace" each nerve at the apex of the axilla. Nerve stimulator can be used as a mean for confirming and identifying nerve localization. For instance, the current to be set between 0.5 and 1 mA to elicit motor response may be useful in this block to identify each nerve. Small volume of LA (5 mL) is injected perineurally to surround each nerve individually. Because of the refractive artifacts, posterior acoustic enhancement of the axillary artery may be mistaken for the radial artery. If identification of each nerve becomes challenging, 20 mL of LA can be injected between the artery and the conjoint tendon to produce an effective block.

Axillary Nerve Block	
Advantages	**Disadvantages**
Superficial block and easy to identify the needle, especially for beginners.	The need to trace each nerve by scanning distally down the arm and using the nerve stimulator to localize each nerve.
Tips and pearls—axillary nerve block	
• If identification of nerves becomes challenging, inject 20 mL of LA above the conjoint tendon will be suffice.	

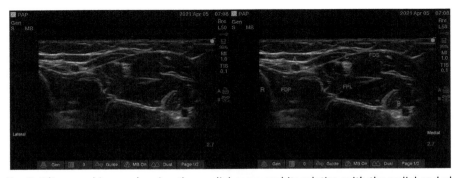

Fig. 6. Ultrasound image showing the medial nerve and its relation with the radial and ulnar artery and nerve in midforearm. (A) Radial artery; (B) ulnar artery and nerve; (C) median nerve radius (FDP, flexor digitorum profundus; FDS, flexor digitorum superficialis; FPL, flexor palmaris longus); (R) radius (FDP, flexor digitorum profundus; FDS, flexor digitorum superficialis; FPL, flexor palmaris longus).

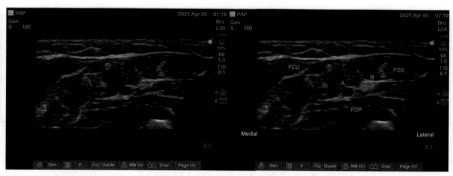

Fig. 7. Ultrasound image showing the ulnar nerve at the forearm. (A) Ulnar artery; (B) ulnar nerve. FCU, flexor carpi ulnaris; FDS, flexor digitorum superficialis; FDP, flexor digitorum profundus; FCU, flexor carpi ulnaris; FDS, flexor digitorum superficialis.

DISTAL BLOCKS OF THE FOREARM

For more distal surgeries, the anesthesiologist can assess the necessary dermatomes and osteotomes required to provide surgical anesthesia. The specific nerves can be targeted individually with small volumes of LA (5 mL).

Median Nerve Block

With the arm placed in the anatomic position, the high-frequency linear transducer (15-6 MHz) is positioned on the forearm. The median nerve can be blocked at the elbow or the forearm, on the medial side of the brachial artery. It can also be traced in the forearm, as it travels in the middle of the tendons (**Fig. 6**) until the carpal tunnel. To limit the risk of nerve injury, it is best to avoid the carpal tunnel area, as the extra pressure from the LA could cause potentially ischemic injury.

Ulnar Nerve Block

With the arm placed in the anatomic position, the high-frequency linear transducer (15–6 MHz) is positioned on the forearm. The ulnar nerve is best blocked at the forearm and not at the elbow, as it is at risk of pressure injury due to its close proximity to the bone. It can be identified easily on the medial aspect of the distal forearm in close proximity to the pulsatile ulnar artery. As the nerve travels proximally, it becomes further away from the artery and can be safely targeted with the nerve block needle (**Fig. 7**).

Radial Nerve Block

With the patient supine or sitting and the arm flexed and positioned on the abdomen, the high-frequency linear transducer (15–6 MHz) is positioned transversely on posterior aspect of the upper arm. The radial nerve can be identified at the midhumerus, as it travels in close proximity to the humerus at the upper arm **Fig. 8**. However, to avoid pressure injury, it should not be blocked at this location; instead the nerve is better blocked at a distal humerus or 2 to 3 cm above the elbow crease before it divides into superficial branch and posterior interosseous branch. The nerve can be traced with the ultrasound transducer initially positioned on the posterior aspect of the upper arm to the anterior aspect at the elbow.

Radial Nerve Block	
Advantages	**Disadvantages**
Easily identifiable, as it can be traced from the humerus distally to the elbow.	Does not have the same duration of anesthesia and analgesia as the more proximal blocks.
Tips and pearls—radial nerve block	
• This block alone does not anesthetize the tourniquet area.	

Pain and Its Negative Effects

Postoperative pain after orthopedic surgeries is one of the most feared surgical complications reported by patients.[7] Poorly controlled acute postoperative pain is predictive of the development of chronic pain.[10] Multimodal analgesic strategies are used to manage acute pain after surgery. The goal is to limit the amount of opioid consumption postoperatively, thus reducing any adverse effects related to their use.[7]

Regional anesthesia is considered to be a cornerstone of the multimodal analgesic approach with numerous advantages such as maximal initial pain control, minimal opioid requirements, and mobilization and rehabilitation in the early perioperative period in patients undergoing orthopedic surgery.[7,11,12]

Recently, rebound pain has gained increased recognition. Rebound pain is defined as quantifiable difference in pain scores when the block is effective versus the increase in pain encountered during the first few hours after the effects or perineural single injection or continuous infusion of local anesthetics.[7] In a retrospective study for patients with wrist fracture surgery, Sunderland and colleagues described an incidence of unplanned physician visits for pain in the first 48 hours of 12% in their single-shot brachial plexus block group, compared with 4% in GA patients.[11] The most important patient-related risk factors associated with the incidence and severity of rebound pain include severe preoperative pain, age less than 60 years, female sex, and psychosocial factors such as pain catastrophizing and depression.[7] The absence of perioperative dexamethasone is also associated with a higher incidence of rebound pain.[13] A defined postdischarge analgesic pathway must be implemented to increase patient satisfaction with their pain management.[11] Multimodal strategies include improved preemptive opioid analgesia during the transition phase before the block completely resolves, the perioperative use of intravenous steroids, better postoperative analgesic pathways and patient education, and the use of adjuvants perineurally or continuous nerve block catheters for several days. The interventions may help reduce the incidence of rebound pain.[7,11] However, a retrospective study by Barry and colleagues showed that despite a high incidence of rebound pain, there were high rates of patient satisfaction with nerve blocks (83.2%), and 96% of patients would choose a PNB again for a future surgery.[13]

ACUTE COMPARTMENT SYNDROME

Acute compartment syndrome (ACS) is a serious complication that occurs most commonly after trauma. ACS results when the pressure within an enclosed compartment increases greater than the capillary perfusion pressure. This compromises the circulation and can lead to muscle ischemia and necrosis.[5,14] The incidence of ACS is 0.25% in distal radius fractures and 3.1% in diaphyseal fractures.[14] The use of regional anesthesia in patients at risk for compartment syndrome is controversial, as most of the literature is based on case reports and expert opinion. However, there is no evidence that peripheral nerve blocks delay the diagnosis of ACS, and most clinicians consider the use of nerve blocks to be safe even in this setting.[5,14,15]

AWAKE OR ASLEEP?

Regional anesthesia can be used as the sole anesthesia technique as well as an adjunct to GA for analgesia purposes. Factors influencing the choice between using sedation or monitored anesthesia care or GA in combination with regional anesthesia include the duration of the surgery, patient positioning for the procedure, and patient preference. Another consideration is the triple bottom line, which takes into consideration the patient, financial, and environmental outcomes. In situations where patients are moribund with multiple comorbidities, the option of regional anesthesia providing surgical anesthesia may be more desirable. There have been studies showing the efficiency of the operating room and financial incentives in patients undergoing regional anesthesia or local anesthesia infiltration for hand surgery.[16,17] Lastly, the reduction in greenhouse gas production by using regional anesthesia and avoiding GA with volatile anesthetics is becoming a greater consideration when discussing global benefits of regional anesthesia.

In cases where a tourniquet is necessary, pain in the upper arm can be managed with sedation with or without ICB nerve block. The ICB, a branch from T2, is a cutaneous sensory nerve that is, spared with a brachial plexus nerve block. The latter can be performed by infiltrating LA subcutaneously just distal to the axilla. In a randomized control trial, the incidence of tourniquet pain was described to be 8.5% and 13.8% under ICB and AXB, respectively. The onset time of pain was 73 to 86 minutes, but no patient required conversion to GA.[18]

For elbow surgeries, the surgical technique sometimes necessitates the patient to be positioned in lateral decubitus or supine position with the flexed arm positioned over the chest or neck area[19]; this can be uncomfortable for the patients, especially if the surgery is prolonged. Therefore, both patient position and surgical duration should be taken into account during discussions about the anesthetic plan. Hand and wrist fracture surgeries are typically shorter in duration, and the patients are positioned supine. Therefore, regional anesthesia with or without sedation can be provided. A notable exception is scaphoid fracture or reconstructive hand surgeries, which tend to be slightly prolonged; therefore, sedation with nerve block catheter consideration may be required.

PERIPHERAL NERVE INJURIES

As it is the case with any technique, brachial plexus blocks are associated with inherent potential risks that are related to either the block placement or toxicity of the medication. The most consequential risk for sport athletes is the potential for debilitating peripheral nerve injury. Although early transient postoperative neurologic symptoms are quite common in the first days to months after PNB, the incidence is reduced with time: 0% to 2.2% at 3 months, 0% to 0.8% at 6 months, and 0% to 0.2% at 1 year. The reported rate of long-term injury is low (2–4 per 10,000 block) and not every peripheral nerve injury (PNI) is block related.[20]

PNIs are classified into 3 categories, from the mildest to severe. Neuropraxia, commonly caused by nerve stretching or compression, is the most frequent. It has a good prognosis, and patients will typically recover full function within weeks to months. Axonotmesis is an axonal injury associated with fascicular impalement, nerve crush, or toxic injury. Recovery following axonal loss can be prolonged and potentially incomplete depending on the intensity of disruption and distance from the injury site.

Proximal axonal lesions are believed to be more severe than more distal lesions (closer to the innervation target). Neurotmesis refers to the complete disruption of the nerve, and prognosis is poor.[21]

The authors' comprehension of PNI is mostly obtained by animal experiments. Mechanisms of PNI related to the use of PNB will fall in one of the three categories: mechanical and injection injury (traumatic injury), vascular or ischemic injury, and chemical or neurotoxic injury.[20,21] Mechanical injuries are caused by forceful needle-nerve contact or by injection into the nerve itself. Intraneural injection may lead to high intraneural pressure, and damage can be done with any type of injectate. Vascular injuries may be secondary to direct injury or acute occlusion of the arteries supplying the nerves. Local anesthetics and adjuncts reduce neural blood flow in a concentration-dependent manner. High-pressure injection can also create neural ischemia. Chemical injuries are caused by tissue toxicity of the injectate. In animal models, most LA can have myotoxic, neurotoxic, and cytotoxic effects in various tissues. There is a direct correlation between concentration of LA and duration of exposure to the nerve and the degree of damage. The site where LA is injected can potentially be the main determinant of neurotoxicity, especially if injection occurs interfascicularly leading to more severe injuries.[7,20,21]

The cause of perioperative PNI is multifactorial. A closed-claim analysis showed that 9 of 53 anesthetic-related brachial plexus injuries were related to intraoperative positioning, and 2 claims were related to regional anesthesia technique.[22] Numerous studies have found that the type of anesthesia (regional vs general) does not influence the incidence of PNI following orthopedic surgeries. However, surgical literature warns that the risk of block-related PNI may be higher than what is reported, and there are anesthetic, patient, and surgical factors that can influence the probabilities.[20,21]

Postoperative neurologic deficits seem more likely related to patient and surgical factors than to PNB. In fact, some patients are at higher risk of PNI, especially if they have preoperative neurologic deficit or compromise, diabetics, or peripheral vascular disease. Specific surgeries also come with their own increased risks, including patient positioning and the use of a tourniquet.[20,21] Anesthetic factors during nerve block performance include intrafascicular injection and direct LA toxicity to the neural tissue, which is time and concentration dependent.[7,20,21]

STRATEGIES TO MITIGATE THE RISK OF NERVE INJURY

Ultrasound is commonly used for PNB; however, its use alone does not eliminate the risk of PNI due to its limitations in resolution and inability to define intraneural versus extraneural injections, even with experts.[23–25] Monitors and additional nerve localization techniques can potentially reduce the risk of PNI, although this remains uncertain.[21,23] Moreover, there are no human data to support the superiority of any single nerve localization technique over another with regard to reducing the likelihood of PNI.[20,21]

The American Association of Regional Anesthesia (ASRA) practice advisory on neurologic complications associated with regional anesthesia states that intraneural needle insertion does not invariably lead to functional nerve injury. However, intrafascicular needle insertion and injection should be avoided. Also, paresthesia during needle advancement or on injection of LA is not entirely predictive of PNI; severe paresthesia should prompt needle repositioning.[20,21] The use of a nerve stimulator alone is not sufficient, because it lacks sensitivity although it is highly specific. Therefore, the absence of motor response does not exclude needle-nerve contact or intraneural nerve placement. However, a positive motor response at 0.2 mA signifies intraneural injection is highly likely.[26] Also, there are no human data to validate the

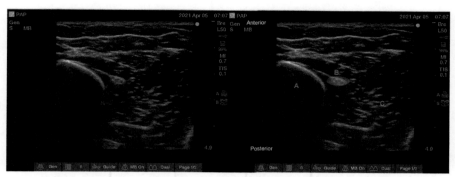

Fig. 8. Ultrasound image showing the radial nerve at the midhumeral level. (A) Humerus; (B) radial nerve; (C) triceps muscle.

effectiveness of injection pressure monitoring for limiting PNI. The common practice of subjectively assessing injection pressure by "hand feel" has been proved inaccurate.[20,21] Although modern ultrasound largely lacks the resolution to detect intraneural injection, when nerve swelling is recognized on the ultrasound, the damage has already been done. With ultrasound, there is a false-negative rate for interpretation of intraneural injection of 16% to 35%.[20,21,27] In a cadaver study for intracluster supraclavicular injection, 24% of subperineural injection was observed with no significant association between sonographic hypoechoic structure expansion and subperineural ink deposits on histology.[28] Furthermore, adequate images of needle-nerve interface are not consistently obtained by all operators and in all patients.[20,21,23,27]

Therefore, a safer approach is to adopt "multimodal monitoring" to minimize intraneural injection. This consists of using multiple monitoring techniques rather than a single modality, which may be unreliable when used alone.[23,27] To avoid forceful needle-nerve contact, needle advancement must ensure that the needle passes through soft tissue layers by applying constant pressure and waiting for the layers to part versus actively advancing the needle within the cluster.[27] In addition to ultrasound visualization, limiting the opening injection pressure (IP) can be beneficial because there is a correlation between high injection pressure and intrafascicular injection. Some devices have been designed to measure the opening IP, and studies have suggested intraneural, in particular, intrafascicular injection, is considered unlikely when opening IP is limited to less than 15 psi.[23,24] Another option to limit the opening IP as well as maintaining low pressure during injection is to apply the compressed air injection technique. It uses a cushion of air above the volume of injectate within a syringe. Therefore, no additional equipment is necessary **Fig. 9**. The air is compressed before transmitting the injection pressure onto the fluid block and less than 50% air compression ensures injection pressures lower than 760 mm Hg.[29] Neurostimulation can be used in combination with ultrasound and injection pressure monitoring to aid with detection of possible needle-nerve contact or intraneural placement.[23] Keeping the stimulation current at 0.2 to 0.5 mA, the needle can be reoriented if a muscle twitch is encountered. Although a safe electrical current threshold cannot be generalized for all, the probability of intraneural or nerve contact is 100% at less than 0.2 mA and close to 50% at 0.5 mA. Using dextrose 5% in water (D5W) for hydrodissection during needle manipulations helps maintain electrical stimulation at the needle tip rather than dispersing the electric current over the shaft of the needle, thus requiring a higher current to elicit a motor response, rendering nerve stimulation uninterpretable. The use of D5W is also somewhat neural protective because it

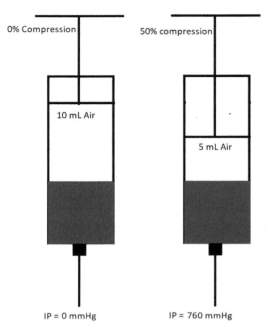

Fig. 9. The use of the compression air injection technique (CAIT) as an objective measurement for the opening injection pressure, as well as for maintaining a low injection pressure throughout the nerve block procedure. IP, injection pressure.

reduces the likelihood of exposing axons to LA while positioning the needle perineurally. Finally, performing the blocks in an awake patient with minimal sedation allows feedback of paresthesia or pain on injection[20,24,27]

LESS IS MORE?

The choice for the optimal nerve block for a specific surgery will ultimately be decided by the anesthesiologist, evaluating the risks and benefits of each technique. One strategy is to limit the duration of nerve tissue exposed to LA, which can potentially cause chemical injury; for instance, opt for single-shot nerve block with lower concentration of LA coupled with good transition pain strategies rather than nerve block infusion. Another consideration may be to avoid tourniquet in patients with a PNB, the use of which can cause pressure injury, resulting in double crush phenomenon.[30–32]

Furthermore, the motto: *primum non nocere*—first do no harm, is relevant especially when providing care to professional athletes where there is limited margin of error and in which a minimalistic approach may be advantageous. Anesthesiologists may decide on blocking only nerves that are absolutely necessary for the surgery (eg, only radial and ulnar nerves for a fifth finger pinning). Proximal axonal lesions are believed to be more severe than more distal lesions (closer to the innervation target). A more proximal nerve lesion on the upper limb has the potential to create an injury involving most of the arm, versus only a single nerve distribution if the injury is more distal.[21] However, there lacks convincing data to confirm or refute the theory that proximal nerve blocks are riskier than more distal approaches.[20]

INFORMED CONSENT

Peripheral nerve injuries are rare and most are transient[20,21]; nonetheless, when they occur, it is devastating for both the patient and the physician. The cause of adverse events is usually multifactorial; therefore, before any nerve block procedure, it is important that informed consent is obtained, outlining risks and benefits as well as alternative options; this should be a routine for all patients because a PNI can affect their livelihood, especially for professional athletes whose prompt recovery of limb function and performance is essential. The most recent reminder of such importance was the $180 million medical malpractice lawsuit filed by a former Minnesota Vikings defensive tackle who suffered an alleged PNI after a nerve block. As regional anesthetists, we have the obligation to inform the risks of PNBs including PNI, chronic pain, or loss of motor function in the blocked limb.

Even if it is considered the standard of care for anesthesia or analgesia for a specific surgery, the athlete must analyze the risks and benefits of undergoing a nerve block compared with alternative pain management techniques in the acute postoperative phase. Ideally, consent should be obtained in advance while patients have the capacity to make an informed choice; this is paramount when the stakes are so high that the patient's career depends on the possible consequences; the decision should not be made under pressure.

CONCLUSION

For upper extremity surgeries, regional anesthetics can be used as an analgesic or anesthetic and have many advantages. The authors have outlined different techniques in anesthetizing the brachial plexus for the elbow, forearm, and hand surgeries. The incidence of peripheral nerve injury related to a nerve block, despite being low, remains present. Surgical, patient, and anesthetic factors can also predispose to nerve injuries. Even though the prevalence is rare, this consequence can ruin a professional athlete's season or even their career. Multimodal monitoring approach is recommended to minimize intraneural injection during nerve blocks. One should consider the risks and benefits carefully when performing nerve blocks on professional athletes, as there is a limited margin of error. A PNI can significantly affect an athlete's livelihood. An open discussion about the risks versus benefits of each technique should occur preoperatively to enable an informed consent to be made for each individual.

SUMMARY

Upper extremity injuries are common among athletes. Regional anesthesia for upper extremity surgeries provides significant benefits and consists of many different brachial plexus approaches. Although there are approaches to ensure safe performance of these nerve blocks, careful balance should be sought in weighing risks and benefits before performing the procedure.

DISCLOSURE

The authors have nothing to disclose.

REFERENCES

1. Sytema R, Dekker R, Dijkstra PU, et al. Upper extremity sports injury: risk factors in comparison to lower extremity injury in more than 25 000 cases. Clin J Sport Med 2010;20(4):256–63.

2. Boyce SH, Quigley MA. Review of sports injuries presenting to an accident and emergency department. Emerg Med J 2004;21(6):704–6.
3. Smucny M, Kolmodin J, Saluan P. Shoulder and elbow injuries in the adolescent athlete. Sports Med Arthrosc Rev 2016;24(4):188–94.
4. Fredericson M, Jennings F, Beaulieu C, et al. Stress fractures in athletes. Top Magn Reson Imaging 2006;17(5):309–25.
5. Gadsden J, Warlick A. Regional anesthesia for the trauma patient: improving patient outcomes. Local Reg Anesth 2015;8:45–55.
6. Dada O, Gonzalez Zacarias A, Ongaigui C, et al. Does rebound pain after peripheral nerve block for orthopedic surgery impact postoperative analgesia and opioid consumption? A narrative review. Int J Environ Res Public Health 2019; 16(18):3257.
7. Tran DQ, Russo G, Muñoz L, et al. A prospective, randomized comparison between ultrasound-guided supraclavicular, infraclavicular, and axillary brachial plexus blocks. Reg Anesth Pain Med 2009;34(4):366–71.
8. Li JW, Songthamwat B, Samy W, et al. Ultrasound-guided costoclavicular brachial plexus block: sonoanatomy, technique, and block dynamics regional. Anesth Pain Med 2017;42:233–40.
9. Horlocker T, Vandermeuelen E, Kopp S, et al. Regional anesthesia in the patient receiving antithrombotic or thrombolytic therapy. American Society of Regional Anesthesia and Pain Medicine Evidence-Based Guideliens (fourth edition). Reg Anesth Pain Med 2018;43:263–309.
10. Gan TJ. Poorly controlled postoperative pain: prevalence, consequences, and prevention. J Pain Res 2017;10:2287–98.
11. Sunderland S, Yarnold CH, Head SJ, et al. Regional versus general anesthesia and the incidence of unplanned health care resource utilization for postoperative pain after wrist fracture surgery: results from a retrospective quality improvement project. Reg Anesth Pain Med 2016;41(1):22–7.
12. Barreveld A, Witte J, Chahal H, et al. Preventive analgesia by local anesthetics: the reduction of postoperative pain by peripheral nerve blocks and intravenous drugs. Anesth Analg 2013;116(5):1141–61.
13. Barry GS, Bailey JG, Sardinha J, et al. Factors associated with rebound pain after peripheral nerve block for ambulatory surgery. Br J Anaesth 2021;126(4):862–71.
14. Mannion S, Capdevila X. Acute compartment syndrome and the role of regional anesthesia. Int Anesthesiol Clin 2010;48(4):85–105.
15. Tran AA, Lee D, Fassihi SC, et al. A systematic review of the effect of regional anesthesia on diagnosis and management of acute compartment syndrome in long bone fractures. Eur J Trauma Emerg Surg 2020;46:1281–90.
16. Holoyda KA, Farhat B, Lalonde DH, et al. Creating an outpatient, local anesthetic hand operating room in a resource-constrained ghanaian hospital builds surgical capacity and financial stability. Ann Plast Surg 2020;84(4):385–9.
17. Wheelock M, Petropolis C, Lalonde DH. The Canadian model for instituting wide-awake hand surgery in our hospitals. Hand Clin 2019;35(1):21–7.
18. Brenner D, Iohom G, Mahon P, et al. George efficacy of axillary versus infraclavicular brachial plexus block in preventing tourniquet pain. Eur J Anaesthesiol 2019; 36(1):48–54.
19. Jennings JD, Hahn A, Rehman S, et al. Management of adult elbow fracture dislocations. Orthop Clin North Am 2016;47(1):97–113.
20. Neal JM, Barrington MJ, Brull R, et al. The second ASRA practice advisory on neurologic complications associated with regional anesthesia and pain medicine: executive summary 2015. Reg Anesth Pain Med 2015;40(5):401–30.

21. Brull R, Hadzic A, Reina MA, et al. Pathophysiology and etiology of nerve injury following peripheral nerve blockade. Reg Anesth Pain Med 2015;40(5):479–90.
22. Kroll DA, Caplan RA, Posner K, et al. Nerve injury associated with anesthesia. Anesthesiology 1990;73:202–7.
23. Varobieff M, Choquet O, Swisser F, et al. Real-time injection pressure sensing and minimal intensity stimulation combination during ultrasound-guided peripheral nerve blocks: an exploratory observational trial. Anesth Analg 2021;132(2):556–65.
24. Ip VHY, Sondekoppam RV, Tsui BC. The scientific principles of multimodal monitoring technique for peripheral nerve blocks: evidence toward a new beginning? Anesth Analg 2021;132(5):e86–8.
25. Krediet AC, Moayeri N, Bleys RL, et al. Intraneural or extraneural: diagnostic accuracy of ultrasound assessment for localizing low-volume injection. Reg Anesth Pain Med 2014;39(5):409–13.
26. Bigeleisen PE, Moayeri N, Groen GJ. Extraneural versus intraneural stimulation thresholds during ultrasound-guided supraclavicular block. Anesthesiology 2009;110:1235–43.
27. Ip VHY, Özelsel TJP, Sondekoppam RV, et al. Multimodal monitoring approach: the key to safe performance of peripheral nerve blocks. Br J Anaesth 2019;123(3):e469–70.
28. Retter S, Szerb J, Kwofie K, et al. Incidence of sub-perineural injection using a targeted intracluster supraclavicular ultrasound-guided approach in cadavers. Br J Anaesth 2019;122(6):776–81.
29. Tsui BC, Li LX, Pillay JJ. Compressed air injection technique to standardize block injection pressures. Can J Anaesth 2006;53:1098–102.
30. Hebl JR, Horlocker TT, Pritchard DJ. Diffuse brachial plexopathy after interscalene blockade in a patient receiving cisplatin chemotherapy: the pharmacologic double crush syndrome. Anesth Analg 2001;92(1):249–51.
31. Molinari WJ 3rd, Elfar JC. The double crush syndrome. J Hand Surg Am 2013;38(4):799–801.
32. Lundborg G, Dahlin LB. The pathophysiology of nerve compression. Hand Clin 1992;8(2):215–27.

Anesthesia for the Patient Undergoing Shoulder Surgery

Jeffrey J. Mojica, DO*, Aaron Ocker, DO, Jaime Barrata, MD,
Eric S. Schwenk, MD

KEYWORDS

- Interscalene block • Beach chair position • Brachial plexus • Peripheral nerve block
- Regional anesthesia • Shoulder surgery

KEY POINTS

- Shoulder surgery can be safely performed either as an inpatient or outpatient procedure and under either general anesthesia or regional anesthesia as the primary anesthetic.
- The interscalene block is the gold standard peripheral nerve block for shoulder surgery, but multiple other alternatives exist.
- The beach chair position is associated with important hemodynamic and physiologic changes.

INTRODUCTION

Shoulder surgery is indicated for degenerative and traumatic injuries involving the glenohumeral joint, acromioclavicular joint, or surrounding structures. Many shoulder pathologies can be surgically repaired with minimally invasive arthroscopic shoulder surgery.[1] In cases of severe disease, a more invasive approach such as total shoulder arthroplasty (TSA) or hemiarthroplasty may be indicated.[2] These procedures have been shown to reduce pain, restore function, and improve the quality of life.[3]

Historically, shoulder surgery was considered an inpatient procedure but improvements in surgical technique, perioperative optimization, blood management, and pain management have led to dramatic reductions in length of stay (LOS).[4] Considering the cost-saving potential, there is significant interest in transitioning shoulder surgery to an outpatient procedure. In this review, we discuss how anesthetic selection, regional anesthesia, and intraoperative positioning are important considerations for the safe delivery of anesthesia in the patient undergoing shoulder surgery.

Department of Anesthesiology, Sidney Kimmel Medical College at Thomas Jefferson University, 111 South 11th Street, Suite 8290 Gibbon Building, Philadelphia, PA 19107, USA
* Corresponding author.
E-mail address: jeffrey.mojica@jefferson.edu

Clin Sports Med 41 (2022) 219–231
https://doi.org/10.1016/j.csm.2021.11.004
0278-5919/22/© 2021 Elsevier Inc. All rights reserved.

SHOULDER ANATOMY

The glenohumeral joint, the surrounding joint capsule, bursae, ligaments, and tendons are innervated by the suprascapular nerve (SSN), axillary nerve, lateral pectoral nerve, musculocutaneous nerve, and subscapular nerves.[5] Each of these nerves arises from the C5 and C6 nerve root and/or originate from the superior trunk of the brachial plexus (**Fig. 1**).[6]

Shoulder arthroplasty involves a surgical incision along the deltopectoral groove, which is innervated by the axillary nerve. Occasionally, the incision has to be extended into the medial arm and axilla into the cutaneous territory of the median cutaneous nerve and intercostobrachial nerves. For arthroscopic shoulder surgery, superior, anterior, lateral, and posterior port-hole incisions are common and correspond to the cutaneous territory of the supraclavicular nerves, axillary nerve, and SSN. The supraclavicular nerves arise from the cervical plexus and provide sensory innervation to the skin above the clavicle (**Fig. 2**).[7]

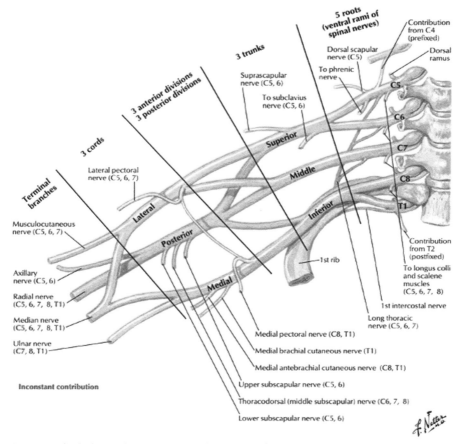

Fig. 1. Brachial plexus. (*From* Limthongthang R, Bachoura A, Songcharoen P, Osterman AL. Adult brachial plexus injury: evaluation and management. Orthop Clin North Am. 2013 Oct;44(4):591-603. doi: 10.1016/j.ocl.2013.06.011. Epub 2013 Sep 6. PMID: 24095074.)

Anterior (palmar) view   **Posterior (dorsal) view**

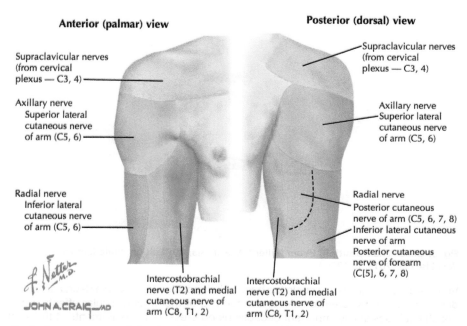

Fig. 2. Sensory nerves of the shoulder. (*From* Anterior (Palmar View): From Netter's Concise Orthopedic Anatomy. Philadelphia, PA: Saunders Elsevier; 2010. p. 98.; and Posterior (Dorsal View): From Netter's Concise Orthopedic Anatomy. Philadelphia, PA: Saunders Elsevier; 2010. p. 99.)

INTRAOPERATIVE ANESTHETIC CONSIDERATIONS
Anesthetic Technique

Shoulder surgery is amenable to either general anesthesia (GA), regional anesthesia, or regional anesthesia with sedation. Of the regional anesthetic techniques, only the interscalene brachial plexus block (ISB) has been shown to consistently produce surgical anesthesia.[8] Hadzic and colleagues studied the impact of anesthetic technique on the quality of the same-day recovery in patients undergoing outpatient rotator cuff surgery.[9] He found that compared with GA alone, patients who received ISB reported less pain, bypassed the postanesthesia care unit more frequently, met discharge criteria more quickly and had no unplanned hospital admissions.[9] Furthermore, patients receiving GA alone were more likely to complain of moderate to severe pain and require unanticipated hospital admission for severe uncontrolled postoperative pain.[9]

INTRAOPERATIVE CHALLENGES RELATED TO POSITIONING

While shoulder surgery can be performed in several patient positions, the beach chair position is commonly used because it provides good access to the shoulder joint (**Fig. 3**). The choice of beach chair versus lateral decubitus position depends on surgeon preference, surgeon experience, and the specific surgery being performed.[10] Advantages of the beach chair position include better anatomic orientation and ability to convert to an open procedure without reprepping.[10] Disadvantages include proximity of endotracheal tube to the surgical field, poor surgical access to the capsulolabral tissue for instability surgery[10] and risk of lateral femoral cutaneous nerve injury.[11]

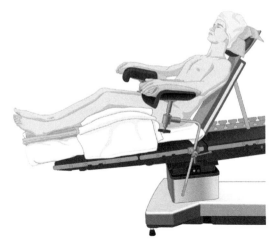

Fig. 3. Beach chair position. (*From* Miller's Anesthesia, 8th Edition. Philadelphia, PA: Saunders Elsevier; 2015. p. 1255.)

Venous pooling can also occur in the beach chair position leading to a decrease in cardiac output and hypotension. An understanding of the cardiovascular effects in the beach chair position is important because blood pressure measurements at the level of the arm do not accurately reflect cerebral perfusion, which can cause brain hypoperfusion and postoperative neurologic events.[12]

Anesthesiologists should be aware of the unique considerations of the beach chair position as it relates to the patient's airway. While some case reports have reported successful outcomes using supraglottic airways,[13] it is the view of the authors that a secure endotracheal tube should be routinely used when GA is selected as the primary anesthetic. The inability of anesthesia providers to access the airway during the case is a major disadvantage and supraglottic airway dislodgments during surgery could necessitate emergent control of the airway in the middle of surgery. The same airway concerns apply to patients that receive sedation and a peripheral nerve block (PNB) as the primary anesthetic technique.

Another potential complication of the beach chair position is lateral femoral cutaneous nerve injury. In one retrospective study, patients with a higher median weight and body mass index were identified as risk factors for lateral femoral cutaneous nerve palsy.[11] Also known as "meralgia paresthetica," this neurologic complication typically presents with paresthesias or dysesthesias in the anterolateral thigh without associated motor weakness.[14] While certainly not a common complication, consideration should be given to counseling obese patients about this risk.

Hypoperfusion to the brain associated with the beach chair position has been a concern for anesthesiologists and surgeons alike for several years.[15] While rare, reports of postoperative vision loss[16] and brain and spinal cord ischemia[17] have surfaced and introduced the question of which patients, if any, should not undergo surgery in the beach chair position. Aguirre and colleagues[12] prospectively studied the effect of the beach chair position on cerebral oxygenation. In their study, regional anesthesia with sedation was used as the primary anesthetic and the authors found that the incidence of cerebral desaturation events was 5%. While no neurologic deficits were detected, patients who experienced such events performed worse on neurobehavioral tests 24 h after surgery. A large database study of 4169 patients, 95.7% of whom received brachial plexus block and sedation, found that no strokes occurred but intraoperative hypotension occurred in almost half.[18] Decreases in mean arterial pressure and middle cerebral artery blood flow velocity have also been observed in patients receiving GA for shoulder surgery in the beach chair position.[19] A retrospective study of 420 shoulder surgery patients detected symptomatic hypotensive/bradycardic events in 61% of patients, 2 of whom had postoperative neurologic complications, and these results led the authors to recommend "proactive hemodynamic management." Several strategies to mitigate brain hypoperfusion have been attempted with limited success. Ko and colleagues[20] compared 2 doses (0.5 mcg/kg/min and 1.0 mcg/kg/min) of intraoperative phenylephrine infusion to placebo during shoulder surgery in beach chair position and found that while the incidence of hypotensive events did not differ among groups, the severity of hypotension was lessened in the high-dose phenylephrine group.

While rare, postoperative stroke has been reported after shoulder surgery in beach chair position[21,22] and the best monitoring and prevention strategies remain unknown. Patients at higher risk for stroke, including those with previous stroke, atrial fibrillation, or carotid artery disease, should be counseled about this risk before surgery or lateral decubitus position could be considered. If invasive blood pressure monitoring is used, the arterial blood pressure transducer should be level with the tragus of the ear to approximate the blood pressure at the Circle of Willis.

For shoulder surgery being performed in the lateral decubitus position, there are also concerns with which the anesthesiologist should be familiar. An obvious challenge is access to the airway if regional anesthesia is the chosen anesthetic technique. Additional concerns include brachial plexus traction injuries,[23] thromboembolic events,[23] and poorer anatomic orientation of anatomy,[10] which could result in longer surgery times or the need to convert to an open procedure with less experienced surgeons.

PERIPHERAL NERVE BLOCKS
Interscalene Block

The ISB is the most widely used PNB for shoulder surgery and can be used as either the primary anesthetic or as an adjunct for postoperative pain management (**Fig. 4**).[24] It has been shown to facilitate hospital discharge by reducing opioid consumption and increasing patient satisfaction, and is recommended for acute postoperative pain management following shoulder surgery.[1]

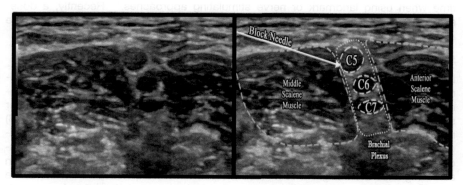

Fig. 4. Interscalene brachial plexus nerve block. The interscalene block targets the C5, C6, and C7 nerve roots of the brachial plexus, which are located between the anterior and middle scalene muscles at the level of the cricoid cartilage.

The primary disadvantage of ISB is the risk of phrenic nerve paralysis and resulting hemidiaphragmatic paralysis (HDP). When large volume injectates ($\geq$20 mLs) are used for ISB, the risk of HDP is approximately 100%.[25] This is due to the proximity of the phrenic nerve to the brachial plexus. Attempts to reduce the incidence of phrenic nerve blockade for ISB, such as ultrasound guidance, reductions in local anesthetic concentration and/or volume, have been unable to reduce the incidence to less than 20%.[8] In the vast majority of patients, phrenic nerve paralysis is transient and resolves with the resolution of analgesia.[26] However, in rare instances, persistent phrenic nerve paralysis can occur. Possible mechanisms of injury include direct needle trauma, inflammatory scarring, or pressure ischemia from high-volume local anesthetics.[26] The most common complaint of phrenic nerve paralysis is dyspnea; however, the vast majority of patients with normal respiratory function do not experience any symptoms.[26] Preexisting lung disease is a relative contraindication to ISB.

Continuous peripheral nerve blocks (CPNBs) are an alternative to single-injection PNBs and can extend the duration of analgesia by delivering a constant infusion of local anesthetic via a perineural catheter. Clinical studies demonstrate continuous interscalene block (CISB) provides superior analgesia, reduces opioid consumption, and opioid-related adverse effects when compared with single-injection ISB.[27] Additional benefits of CISB include improved sleep, improved patient satisfaction, reduction in postoperative nausea and vomiting (PONV), and less dynamic and resting pain for up to 48 hours after major shoulder surgery.[27] Perineural catheters can be attached to ambulatory infusion pumps and can deliver 72 hours or longer of pain relief after hospital discharge.

Adverse effects of ISB include HDP, vascular puncture, Horner's syndrome, and hoarseness due to unilateral recurrent laryngeal nerve blockade.[7] Complications of CPNBs include secondary block failure, perineural catheter migration, dislodgement or obstruction, fluid leakage at the catheter site, infusion pump malfunctions, and local anesthetic systemic toxicity.

Supraclavicular Block

The supraclavicular block anesthetizes the divisions of the brachial plexus at the supraclavicular fossa. Compared with ISB, the supraclavicular block provides comparable levels of analgesia, opioid consumption, and patient satisfaction, but with a lower incidence of adverse effects for shoulder surgery.[28] The incidence of HDP for supraclavicular block is significantly less than the ISB, but still occurs 50% of the time when using landmark or nerve stimulating approaches.[29] Recently, a dose-escalation study demonstrated a 33% incidence of HDP, despite ultrasound guidance and an injectate volume of 5 mL.[30]

Suprascapular Nerve Block

Despite the success of the ISB, concerns regarding its safety and its effects on respiratory function have led to the development of alternative regional anesthetic techniques. As the SSN is believed to transmit most of the pain following shoulder surgery, it was hypothesized that an isolated suprascapular nerve block (SSNB) may be sufficient for postoperative analgesia. The SSN can be anesthetized posteriorly at the supraspinous fossa[31] or anteriorly as it courses beneath the omohyoid muscle.[32] Cadaveric studies indicate that the anterior approach may be more effective in achieving shoulder analgesia as it reliably anesthetizes the proximal branches of the SSN,[32] which are spared when the nerve is blocked posteriorly.[33] In a large multicenter randomized controlled trial (RCT), the anterior SSNB was shown to provide noninferior analgesia to the ISB in patients undergoing arthroscopic shoulder surgery.[34] The mechanism of analgesia was attributed to indirect blockade of the superior trunk of the brachial plexus and was based on the motor and sensory assessment of isolated C5 and C6 functions.[34]

Combined Posterior Suprascapular and Axillary Nerve Block

Price suggested supplementing the posterior SSNB with a selective axillary nerve block as a way to improve the quality of analgesia.[35] The combined posterior SSNB and axillary nerve block has been shown to reduce postoperative pain scores for arthroscopic rotator cuff repair when compared with the posterior SSNB alone.[36] However, this approach does not compare favorably when compared with the ISB.[37] Thus, while the combined posterior SSNB and axillary nerve block may be beneficial for minor shoulder surgery, it is likely to be insufficient for major shoulder surgery.[8]

Combined Anterior Suprascapular and Infraclavicular Nerve Block

The SSNB anesthetizes the posterior shoulder and the infraclavicular block anesthetizes the anterior shoulder by targeting the nerves that arise from the posterior and lateral cord. Theoretically, this combination would anesthetize most of the nerves that innervate the shoulder.[38] Taha and colleagues were one of the first groups to study this technique and found it to be comparable to a low-volume ISB in terms of duration of analgesia, morphine consumption, and patient satisfaction.[39] Furthermore, the combined SSNB and infraclavicular approach better preserved diaphragmatic function, suggesting a role in patients with respiratory contraindications to ISB.[39]

Superior Trunk Block

The superior trunk block (STB) was described as an alternative to the ISB with phrenic-nerve sparing potential.[40] As many of the nerves that innervate the shoulder arise from the superior trunk, a smaller volume of local anesthetic may be sufficient to produce shoulder analgesia, and may also spare the phrenic nerve. Clinical studies demonstrate that an STB using 15 mL of local anesthetic produces noninferior analgesia to ISB for arthroscopic shoulder surgery, but with a lower rate of HDP.[6,41]

Costoclavicular Block

The costoclavicular block (CCB) targets the brachial plexus in the costoclavicular space (CCS).[42] Aliste and colleagues speculated that local anesthetic injected into the CCS could produce comparable levels of analgesia by serving as a "retrograde channel to the supraclavicular brachial plexus [and] suprascapular nerve." The authors hoped that this approach could also spare the phrenic nerve.[43] In an RCT comparing the CCB and the ISB for arthroscopic shoulder surgery, the authors found no statistical difference between the 2 groups in terms of pain scores, intra and postoperative opioid consumption, opioid-related adverse effects, and patient satisfaction.[43] Interestingly, none of the 22 patients in the CCB group had evidence of HDP, compared with 100% of the ISB group.[43]

ROLE OF LIPOSOMAL BUPIVACAINE AND OTHER ADDITIVES

Liposomal bupivacaine (LB) (Pacira BioSciences, Parsippany, NJ, USA) is an injectable suspension that uses a lipid-based delivery system releasing multivesicular liposomal particles more than a 72-h time period and purports to produce approximately 24 to 72 hours of analgesia.[44] It was approved by the U.S. Food and Drug Administration (FDA) in 2018 for both local infiltration analgesia (LIA) and for interscalene perineural injection.[45]

Overall, neither perineural LB nor LIA with LB seem to confer advantages over non-liposomal local anesthetics in terms of pain relief, opioid consumption, or opioid-related adverse effects.[46] In fact, some studies demonstrated that LIA with LB was associated with an increase in pain and opioid consumption in the immediate postoperative period when compared with single-injection ISB[47] or continuous ISB[48] following shoulder surgery.

Several local anesthetic additives have been incorporated into ISB, and although they are widely used in clinical practice, they are not approved for perineural use by the FDA. Dexamethasone is one of the most widely studied local anesthetic additives for PNBs, but considerable debate remains regarding the optimal route and dose of administration. Cummings and colleagues demonstrated the duration of analgesia for ISB could be extended more than 22 hours by adding 8 mg of perineural dexamethasone to either bupivacaine or ropivacaine.[49] The block prolongation effect has been shown to persist at lower doses of 1 mg, 2 mg, and 4 mg.[50,51]

Similarly, intravenous (IV) dexamethasone doses of 4 mg and 10 mg have also been shown to increase the duration of ISB.[52] In a meta-analysis comparing the effect of perineural and IV dexamethasone in PNBs, perineural dexamethasone was found to prolong block duration by 3.77 hours and decrease opioid consumption at 24 hours when compared with IV dexamethasone.[53] However, the authors cautioned that perineural dexamethasone is off-label and any advantages must be weighed against the unknown long-term risks of perineural administration.[53]

Other local anesthetic additives that are used to increase the duration of PNB include epinephrine, dexmedetomidine, and buprenorphine. Epinephrine results in block prolongation secondary to local vasoconstriction and reduced systemic absorption. The effects of epinephrine are more pronounced for short-acting local anesthetics such as lidocaine and mepivacaine and provide little to no benefit when added to long-acting local anesthetics.[54] Perineural doses between 50 and 60 mcg of dexmedetomidine can prolong sensory blockade, increase block onset, and reduced opioid consumption with minimal hemodynamic effects.[55] Although perineural buprenorphine can prolong the duration of PNB, it is associated with a significant increase in PONV.[56]

SUMMARY

Shoulder surgery presents several challenges for the anesthesiologist. Regional anesthesia techniques provide superior analgesia than opioids alone and should be used whenever possible for most patients undergoing should surgery. The interscalene block is the gold standard for analgesia after shoulder surgery but comes with a consistent risk of phrenic nerve blockade. Alternative PNBs, including combinations of blocks, may be chosen for patients with compromised respiratory function to reduce the risk of phrenic nerve blockade. Continuous catheter techniques can extend the duration of analgesia if desired. LB does not have consistent evidence supporting it over plain bupivacaine for PNBs. Finally, patient positioning during shoulder surgery introduces several risks including nerve traction injuries and ischemic events of the central nervous system that can be devastating. The optimal mitigation strategy remains unknown but some patients may not be good candidates for beach chair position and hypotension should be aggressively treated and prevented if possible.

CLINICS CARE POINTS

- Shoulder surgery can be safely performed in the outpatient setting using general anesthesia or regional anesthesia as the primary anesthetic.

- Multimodal analgesia with non-opioid analgesics and regional anesthesia is recommended for postoperative analgesia following shoulder surgery.
- The interscalene nerve block is the gold-standard peripheral nerve block, whose main disadvantage is diaphragmatic hemiparesis; fortunately, there are many alternative nerve blocks that can provide comparable levels of analgesia.

DISCLOSURE

The authors have no relevant disclosures, conflicts of interest, or funding to declare for this article.

REFERENCES

1. Warrender WJ, Syed UAM, Hammoud S, et al. Pain management after outpatient shoulder arthroscopy: a systematic review of randomized controlled trials. Am J Sports Med 2017;45(7):1676–86. https://doi.org/10.1177/0363546516667906.
2. Ahmed AF, Hantouly A, Toubasi A, et al. The safety of outpatient total shoulder arthroplasty: a systematic review and meta-analysis. Int Orthop 2021;45(3): 697–710. https://doi.org/10.1007/s00264-021-04940-7.
3. Carter MJ, Mikuls TR, Nayak S, et al. Impact of total shoulder arthroplasty on generic and shoulder-specific health-related quality-of-life measures: a systematic literature review and meta-analysis. J Bone Joint Surg Am 2012;94(17): e127. https://doi.org/10.2106/JBJS.K.00204.
4. Brolin TJ, Mulligan RP, Azar FM, et al. Neer Award 2016: outpatient total shoulder arthroplasty in an ambulatory surgery center is a safe alternative to inpatient total shoulder arthroplasty in a hospital: a matched cohort study. J Shoulder Elbow Surg 2017;26(2):204–8. https://doi.org/10.1016/j.jse.2016.07.011.
5. Tran J, Peng PWH, Agur AMR. Anatomical study of the innervation of glenohumeral and acromioclavicular joint capsules: implications for image-guided intervention. Reg Anesth Pain Med 2019;44(4):452–8. https://doi.org/10.1136/rapm-2018-100152.
6. Kim DH, Lin Y, Beathe JC, et al. Superior trunk block. Anesthesiology 2019; 131(3):521–33. https://doi.org/10.1097/aln.0000000000002841.
7. Neal JM, Gerancher JC, Hebl JR, et al. Upper extremity regional anesthesia. Reg Anesth Pain Med 2009;34(2):134–70. https://doi.org/10.1097/aap. 0b013e31819624eb.
8. Tran DQH, Elgueta MF, Aliste J, et al. Diaphragm-sparing nerve blocks for shoulder surgery. Reg Anesth Pain Med 2017;42(1):32–8. https://doi.org/10.1097/aap. 0000000000000529.
9. Hadzic A, Williams A, Brian, et al. For outpatient rotator cuff surgery, nerve block anesthesia provides superior same-day recovery over general anesthesia. Anesthesiology 2005;102(5):1001–7. https://doi.org/10.1097/00000542-200505000-00020.
10. Keyurapan E, Chuaychoosakoon C. Modified semilateral decubitus position for shoulder arthroscopy and its application for open surgery of the shoulder (one setting for all shoulder procedures). Arthrosc Tech 2018;7(4):e307–12. https://doi.org/10.1016/j.eats.2017.09.008.
11. Holtzman AJ, Glezos CD, Feit EJ, et al. Prevalence and risk factors for lateral femoral cutaneous nerve palsy in the beach chair position. Arthroscopy 2017; 33(11):1958–62. https://doi.org/10.1016/j.arthro.2017.06.050.

12. Aguirre JA, Marzendorfer O, Brada M, et al. Cerebral oxygenation in the beach chair position for shoulder surgery in regional anesthesia: impact on cerebral blood flow and neurobehavioral outcome. J Clin Anesth 2016;35:456–64. https://doi.org/10.1016/j.jclinane.2016.08.035.

13. Tan LZ, Tan DJA, Seet E. Use of the Laryngeal Mask Airway (LMA) protector for shoulder surgeries in beach-chair position. J Clin Anesth 2017;39:110–1. https://doi.org/10.1016/j.jclinane.2017.03.036.

14. Fargo MV, Konitzer LN. Meralgia paresthetica due to body armor wear in U.S. soldiers serving in Iraq: a case report and review of the literature. Mil Med 2007; 172(6):663–5. https://doi.org/10.7205/milmed.172.6.663.

15. Papadonikolakis A, Wiesler ER, Olympio MA, et al. Avoiding catastrophic complications of stroke and death related to shoulder surgery in the sitting position. Arthroscopy 2008;24(4):481–2. https://doi.org/10.1016/j.arthro.2008.02.005.

16. Bhatti MT, Enneking FK. Visual loss and ophthalmoplegia after shoulder surgery. Anesth Analg 2003;96(3):899–902. https://doi.org/10.1213/01.ane.0000047272. 31849.f9, table of contents.

17. Pohl A, Cullen DJ. Cerebral ischemia during shoulder surgery in the upright position: a case series. J Clin Anesth 2005;17(6):463–9. https://doi.org/10.1016/j. jclinane.2004.09.012.

18. Yadeau JT, Casciano M, Liu SS, et al. Stroke, regional anesthesia in the sitting position, and hypotension: a review of 4169 ambulatory surgery patients. Reg Anesth Pain Med 2011;36(5):430–5. https://doi.org/10.1097/AAP.0b013e318228d54e.

19. Hanouz JL, Fiant AL, Gerard JL. Middle cerebral artery blood flow velocity during beach chair position for shoulder surgery under general anesthesia. J Clin Anesth 2016;33:31–6. https://doi.org/10.1016/j.jclinane.2016.01.009.

20. Ko MJ, Kim H, Lee HS, et al. Effect of phenylephrine infusion on hypotension induced by the beach chair position: a prospective randomized trial. Medicine (Baltimore) 2020;99(28):e20946. https://doi.org/10.1097/MD.0000000000020946.

21. van Erp JHJ, Ostendorf M, Lansdaal JR. Shoulder surgery in beach chair position causing perioperative stroke: four cases and a review of the literature. J Orthop 2019;16(6):493–5. https://doi.org/10.1016/j.jor.2019.05.009.

22. Kent CD, Stephens LS, Posner KL, et al. What adverse events and injuries are cited in anesthesia malpractice claims for nonspine orthopaedic surgery? Clin Orthop Relat Res 2017;475(12):2941–51. https://doi.org/10.1007/s11999-017-5303-z.

23. Li X, Eichinger JK, Hartshorn T, et al. A comparison of the lateral decubitus and beach-chair positions for shoulder surgery: advantages and complications. J Am Acad Orthop Surg 2015;23(1):18–28. https://doi.org/10.5435/JAAOS-23-01-18.

24. Chan JJ, Cirino CM, Vargas L, et al. Peripheral nerve block use in inpatient and outpatient shoulder arthroplasty: a population-based study evaluating utilization and outcomes. Reg Anesth Pain Med 2020;45(10):818–25. https://doi.org/10. 1136/rapm-2020-101522.

25. Urmey WF, Talts KH, Sharrock NE. One hundred percent incidence of hemidiaphragmatic paresis associated with interscalene brachial plexus anesthesia as diagnosed by ultrasonography. Anesth Analg 1991;72(4):498–503. https://doi. org/10.1213/00000539-199104000-00014.

26. El-Boghdadly K, Chin KJ, Chan VWS. Phrenic nerve palsy and regional anesthesia for shoulder surgery. Anesthesiology 2017;127(1):173–91. https://doi.org/ 10.1097/aln.0000000000001668.

27. Ilfeld BM, Morey TE, Wright TW, et al. Continuous interscalene brachial plexus block for postoperative pain control at home: a randomized, double-blinded,

placebo-controlled study. Anesth Analg 2003;96(4):1089–95. https://doi.org/10.1213/01.ane.0000049824.51036.ef.

28. Auyong DB, Yuan SC, Choi DS, et al. A double-blind randomized comparison of continuous interscalene, supraclavicular, and suprascapular blocks for total shoulder arthroplasty. Reg Anesth Pain Med 2017;42(3):302–9. https://doi.org/10.1097/AAP.0000000000000578.

29. Neal JM, Moore JM, Kopacz DJ, et al. Quantitative analysis of respiratory, motor, and sensory function after supraclavicular block. Anesth Analg 1998;86(6):1239–44. https://doi.org/10.1097/00000539-199806000-00020.

30. Tedore TR, Lin HX, Pryor KO, et al. Dose–response relationship between local anesthetic volume and hemidiaphragmatic paresis following ultrasound-guided supraclavicular brachial plexus blockade. Reg Anesth Pain Med 2020;45(12):979–84. https://doi.org/10.1136/rapm-2020-101728.

31. Chan CW, Peng PW. Suprascapular nerve block: a narrative review. Reg Anesth Pain Med 2011;36(4):358–73. https://doi.org/10.1097/AAP.0b013e3182204ec0.

32. Siegenthaler A, Moriggl B, Mlekusch S, et al. Ultrasound-guided suprascapular nerve block, description of a novel supraclavicular approach. Reg Anesth Pain Med 2012;37(3):325–8. https://doi.org/10.1097/aap.0b013e3182409168.

33. Eckmann MS, Bickelhaupt B, Fehl J, et al. Cadaveric study of the articular branches of the shoulder joint. Reg Anesth Pain Med 2017;42(5):564–70. https://doi.org/10.1097/AAP.0000000000000652.

34. Abdallah FW, Wijeysundera DN, Laupacis A, et al. Subomohyoid anterior suprascapular block versus interscalene block for arthroscopic shoulder surgery: a multicenter randomized trial. Anesthesiology 2020;132(4):839–53. https://doi.org/10.1097/ALN.0000000000003132.

35. Price DJ. The shoulder block: a new alternative to interscalene brachial plexus blockade for the control of postoperative shoulder pain. Anaesth Intensive Care 2007;35(4):575–81. https://doi.org/10.1177/0310057x0703500418.

36. Lee JJ, Kim DY, Hwang JT, et al. Effect of ultrasonographically guided axillary nerve block combined with suprascapular nerve block in arthroscopic rotator cuff repair: a randomized controlled trial. Arthroscopy 2014;30(8):906–14. https://doi.org/10.1016/j.arthro.2014.03.014.

37. Pani N, Routray SS, Pani S, et al. Post-operative analgesia for shoulder arthroscopic surgeries: a comparison between inter-scalene block and shoulder block. Indian J Anaesth 2019;63(5):382–7. https://doi.org/10.4103/ija.IJA_65_19.

38. Tran DQ, Layera S, Bravo D, et al. Diaphragm-sparing nerve blocks for shoulder surgery, revisited. Reg Anesth Pain Med 2020;45(1):73–8. https://doi.org/10.1136/rapm-2019-100908.

39. Taha AM, Yurdi NA, Elahl MI, et al. Diaphragm-sparing effect of the infraclavicular subomohyoid block vs low volume interscalene block. A randomized blinded study. Acta Anaesthesiol Scand 2019;63(5):653–8. https://doi.org/10.1111/aas.13322.

40. Burckett-St Laurent D, Chan V, Chin KJ. Refining the ultrasound-guided interscalene brachial plexus block: the superior trunk approach. Can J Anaesth 2014;61(12):1098–102. https://doi.org/10.1007/s12630-014-0237-3.

41. Kang R, Jeong JS, Chin KJ, et al. Superior trunk block provides noninferior analgesia compared with interscalene brachial plexus block in arthroscopic shoulder surgery. Anesthesiology 2019;131(6):1316–26. https://doi.org/10.1097/aln.0000000000002919.

42. Karmakar MK, Sala-Blanch X, Songthamwat B, et al. Benefits of the costoclavicular space for ultrasound-guided infraclavicular brachial plexus block:

description of a costoclavicular approach. Reg Anesth Pain Med 2015;40(3): 287–8. https://doi.org/10.1097/AAP.0000000000000232.

43. Aliste J, Bravo D, Layera S, et al. Randomized comparison between interscalene and costoclavicular blocks for arthroscopic shoulder surgery. Reg Anesth Pain Med 2019;44(4):472–7. https://doi.org/10.1136/rapm-2018-100055.

44. Chahar P, Cummings KC 3rd. Liposomal bupivacaine: a review of a new bupivacaine formulation. J Pain Res 2012;5:257–64. https://doi.org/10.2147/jpr.S27894.

45. U. S. Food and Drug Administration. FDA in brief: FDA approves new use of exparel for nerve block pain relief following shoulder surgeries. Available at: https://www.fda.gov/news-events/fda-brief/fda-brief-fda-approves-new-use-exparel-nerve-block-pain-relief-following-shoulder-surgeries. Accessed July 13, 2021.

46. Kolade O, Patel K, Ihejirika R, et al. Efficacy of liposomal bupivacaine in shoulder surgery: a systematic review and meta-analysis. J Shoulder Elbow Surg 2019; 28(9):1824–34. https://doi.org/10.1016/j.jse.2019.04.054.

47. Namdari S, Nicholson T, Abboud J, et al. Randomized controlled trial of interscalene block compared with injectable liposomal bupivacaine in shoulder arthroplasty. J Bone Joint Surg Am 2017;99(7):550–6. https://doi.org/10.2106/jbjs.16.00296.

48. Abildgaard JT, Lonergan KT, Tolan SJ, et al. Liposomal bupivacaine versus indwelling interscalene nerve block for postoperative pain control in shoulder arthroplasty: a prospective randomized controlled trial. J Shoulder Elbow Surg 2017;26(7):1175–81. https://doi.org/10.1016/j.jse.2017.03.012.

49. Cummings KC 3rd, Napierkowski DE, Parra-Sanchez I, et al. Effect of dexamethasone on the duration of interscalene nerve blocks with ropivacaine or bupivacaine. Br J Anaesth 2011;107(3):446–53. https://doi.org/10.1093/bja/aer159.

50. Holland D, Amadeo RJJ, Wolfe S, et al. Effect of dexamethasone dose and route on the duration of interscalene brachial plexus block for outpatient arthroscopic shoulder surgery: a randomized controlled trial. [Effet de la dose et de la voie d'administration de la dexaméthasone sur la durée d'un bloc interscalénique du plexus brachial pour l'arthroscopie de l'épaule réalisée en chirurgie ambulatoire: une étude randomisée contrôlée]. Can J Anaesth 2018;65(1):34–45. https://doi.org/10.1007/s12630-017-0989-7.

51. Gouda N, Zangrilli J, Voskerijian A, et al. Safety and duration of low-dose adjuvant dexamethasone in regional anesthesia for upper extremity surgery: a prospective, randomized, controlled blinded study. Hand (N Y) 2021. https://doi.org/10.1177/15589447211008558.

52. Chalifoux F, Colin F, St-Pierre P, et al. Low dose intravenous dexamethasone (4 mg and 10 mg) significantly prolongs the analgesic duration of single-shot interscalene block after arthroscopic shoulder surgery: a prospective randomized placebo-controlled study. [La dexamethasone intraveineuse a des doses de 4 mg ou de 10 mg prolonge significativement la duree analgesique du bloc interscalenique simple suite a une chirurgie arthroscopique de l'epaule: une etude prospective, randomisee et controlee avec placebo]. Can J Anaesth 2017; 64(3):280–9. https://doi.org/10.1007/s12630-016-0796-6.

53. Chong MA, Berbenetz NM, Lin C, et al. Perineural versus intravenous dexamethasone as an adjuvant for peripheral nerve blocks: a systematic review and meta-analysis. Reg Anesth Pain Med 2017;42(3):319–26. https://doi.org/10.1097/aap.0000000000000571.

54. Schoenmakers KP, Fenten MG, Louwerens JW, et al. The effects of adding epinephrine to ropivacaine for popliteal nerve block on the duration of postoperative analgesia: a randomized controlled trial. BMC Anesthesiol 2015;15:100. https://doi.org/10.1186/s12871-015-0083-z.

55. Vorobeichik L, Brull R, Abdallah FW. Evidence basis for using perineural dexme-detomidine to enhance the quality of brachial plexus nerve blocks: a systematic review and meta-analysis of randomized controlled trials. Br J Anaesth 2017; 118(2):167–81. https://doi.org/10.1093/bja/aew411.

56. Schnabel A, Reichl SU, Zahn PK, et al. Efficacy and safety of buprenorphine in peripheral nerve blocks: a meta-analysis of randomised controlled trials. Eur J Anaesthesiol 2017;34(9):576–86. https://doi.org/10.1097/eja.0000000000000628.

Regional Anesthesia for Hip Arthroscopy

Peter E. Amato, MD[a],*, Andrew J. Winkelman, BS[b], Grace L. Forster, BS[b], F. Winston Gwathmey Jr, MD[c]

KEYWORDS

- Hip arthroscopy • Regional anesthesia • Analgesia • Anatomy • Nerve blocks

KEY POINTS

- Hip arthroscopy can be painful, and many narcotic-sparing analgesic strategies have been used, but none are uniformly effective.
- The sensory innervation of the hip joint is complex, with input from the femoral, obturator, accessory obturator, sciatic, superior and inferior gluteal nerves, and the nerve to the quadratus femoris.
- Regional nerve blocks may provide some degree of analgesia, but many cause lower extremity weakness and can lead to falls.
- Local infiltration techniques may provide some degree of analgesia, but none are exceptional.
- Newer ultrasound-guided fascial plane blocks have potential for motor sparing analgesia, but require further investigation.

INTRODUCTION

Over the last decade, hip arthroscopy has become a more common outpatient surgical procedure, increasing in incidence by 365%.[1] The spectrum of indications has broadened, including femoroacetabular impingement (FAI), labral injury, chondral damage, loose bodies, osteoarthritis, snapping hip syndromes, trochanteric pain, and iliopsoas and gluteal tendon tears. With ongoing improvements in technique and training, we can expect the prevalence of cases to continue to increase, underscoring the need for reliable pain management.

---

[a] Acute Pain Service, Department of Anesthesiology, University of Virginia Health System, University of Virginia, PO Box 800710, Charlottesville, VA 22908-0710, USA; [b] Department of Anesthesiology, University of Virginia Health System, University of Virginia, PO Box 800710, Charlottesville, VA 22908-0710, USA; [c] Department of Orthopaedic Surgery, University of Virginia Health System, University of Virginia, 515 Ray C. Hunt Drive, Charlottesville, VA, 22908 USA
* Corresponding author.
E-mail address: pea2m@hscmail.mcc.virginia.edu

Clin Sports Med 41 (2022) 233–246
https://doi.org/10.1016/j.csm.2021.11.001
0278-5919/22/© 2021 Elsevier Inc. All rights reserved.

Pain after hip arthroscopy may be severe[2] and currently requires the use of opioid medications for some period postoperatively. A recent study reported an average total narcotic consumption of 91 mg of oxycodone over the first 9 postoperative days (PODs), with the highest daily consumption occurring early in the study period.[3] Pain and sequelae of opioid therapy such as gastrointestinal complaints, occupy the top 2 most common causes for emergency department visits after hip arthroscopy,[4] and represent significant causes of unplanned admission from ambulatory surgery centers on the day of surgery.[5] The associated health care costs are significant, and these events contribute to poor patient satisfaction. An optimal narcotic-sparing analgesic strategy for the perioperative period is obviously needed, yet still eludes us.

This article begins by reviewing elements of the surgical procedure and sensory innervation relevant to the most common hip arthroscopic procedures, followed by an evidence-based review of existing local anesthetic-based injection techniques. Blinded, randomized control trials were sought whenever possible. Although this topic has been reviewed before, newer motor-sparing fascial plane blocks now exist, which may offer greater simplicity and safety.

PROCEDURE AND ANATOMY

External landmarks to place arthroscopic portals include the anterior superior iliac spine (ASIS) and the tip of the greater trochanter (GT). The "safe zone" for hip arthroscopy is lateral to the line running distally from the ASIS to the patella.[6] This zone avoids injury to the femoral neurovascular bundle. Arthroscopic access to the hip joint is performed through a combination of 2 to 5 portals depending on the procedure (**Fig. 1**). After traction is applied, the anterolateral (AL) portal is generally the first portal placed.

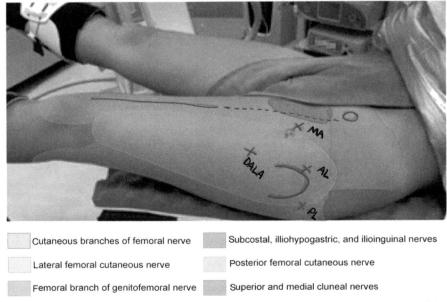

Cutaneous branches of femoral nerve	Subcostal, illiohypogastric, and ilioinguinal nerves
Lateral femoral cutaneous nerve	Posterior femoral cutaneous nerve
Femoral branch of genitofemoral nerve	Superior and medial cluneal nerves

Fig. 1. Left hip with portal sites marked and overlying cutaneous nerve map. Curved line represents GT; circle represents ASIS; straight and dotted lines are drawn from ASIS to patella. Lateral to this marks the "safe zone." AL, anterolateral portal; DALA, distal anterolateral accessory portal; MA, midanterior portal; PL, posterolateral portal.

This is located 1 cm proximal and slightly anterior to the tip of the GT, and fluoroscopy is used to localize proper placement in the joint. The second portal placed is an anterior portal. Historically, this portal was placed at the intersection of the line extending distally from the ASIS and medially from the tip of the GT. A midanterior (MA) portal lateral and distal to the conventional anterior portal has been described to decrease risk to the lateral femoral cutaneous nerve (LFCN) and improve access to the joint. Accessory portals include a distal anterolateral accessory portal (DALA) and posterolateral (PL) portal. Other portals can be used within the safe zone for instrumentation and suture management.

The LFCN is the most commonly injured nerve during hip arthroscopy. This nerve exits the pelvis deep to the inguinal ligament approximately 1 cm medial to the ASIS and runs on the fascia of the sartorius muscle before dividing into an anterior and posterior division. The anterior division exits the fascia more distally to provide cutaneous sensation to the distal AL thigh, whereas the posterior division provides sensation more proximally in the area of the GT and proximal lateral thigh. Most portals will pass through skin innervated by the LFCN (see **Fig. 1**), and thoughtful placement may reduce the risk of piercing a large branch. Depending on exact placement, portals could pass through cutaneous regions of the femoral nerve (FN) medially, posterior femoral cutaneous nerve posteriorly, or more superiorly through other lumbar plexus territories.

Most corrective FAI procedures involve entering the anterior and superior capsule to reduce femoral and acetabular areas of impingement. Labral tears associated with FAI more commonly occur in the anterior and anterior superior regions as well.[7] The sensory innervation of the joint is complex, and has been the subject of multiple anatomic studies and reviews.[8–11]

The anterior surfaces of the joint receive articular branches from the femoral, obturator, and accessory obturator nerves. In a cadaveric study, Short and colleagues[10] found that both the FN and obturator nerve (ON) were found in all anatomic specimens examined, whereas the accessory obturator nerve (AON) was found in only 53.8%. Both the FN and AON branches descended toward the joint between the anterior inferior iliac spine and the iliopubic eminence, whereas the ON branches passed close to the inferomedial acetabulum. The FN supplied the superolateral and inferolateral portions of the anterior joint in most cases, with fewer specimens showing superomedial supply. The ON was found to reach the inferomedial and inferolateral portions, whereas the accessory obturator supplied the superomedial and inferomedial regions when present (**Fig. 2**). The greatest density of nerve fibers appears to be in the superolateral capsule;[12] however, the clinical significance of how this relates to nociception is unclear. The labrum has also been studied, with dense sensory innervation found in the anterosuperior and posterosuperior regions,[13,14] with high concentrations at the labral-acetabular junction.[15]

Articular branches to the posterior joint include those from the sciatic, superior gluteal, inferior gluteal, and quadratus femoris nerves. Compared with the anterior joint, this region appears to be more variable, with fewer studies available for review. Kampa and colleagues[16] were able to identify articular branches with greater frequency across specimens compared with previous anatomic studies. The most frequently identified branches were those from the nerve to the quadratus femoris (100%), primarily found in the inferomedial capsule. Sciatic nerve fibers were visible in 85% of dissections, most often contributing to the superomedial capsule. A similar rate of superior gluteal nerve involvement was found, most often reaching the superolateral joint, overlapping with the sciatic regions. The inferior gluteal nerve probably contributes the least to sensation, as it was infrequently found innervating the posteroinferior capsule. **Fig. 3** shows the location of the posterior articular branches.

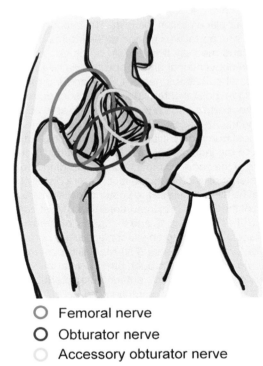

○ Femoral nerve
○ Obturator nerve
○ Accessory obturator nerve

Fig. 2. Innervation of the anterior hip joint. Colored circles represent portions of the capsule and joint innervated by the femoral (*red*), obturator (*blue*), and accessory obturator nerves (*yellow*).

Impingement correction involves burring of the femoral head and/or acetabulum, the extent of which may contribute significantly to the magnitude of postoperative pain.[17] Our understanding of the underlying periosteal sensory innervation generally follows the patterns described earlier for the surrounding capsule. Most of the anterior femoral head is supplied by FN branches. The medial surface is largely obturator, and the PL side is innervated by a mix of sacral plexus nerves.

A final aspect of hip arthroscopy that deserves attention is the frequent extravasation of fluid outside the joint. Although clinical sequelae are rare, as much as 10% of total arthroscopic fluid volume can track to the thigh, gluteus, peritoneum, and retroperitoneum during routine cases studied with computed tomography scans.[18] Fluid collections can be identified postoperatively by FAST (Focused Assessment with Sonography for Trauma) examination, and are associated with greater postoperative pain.[19] Extravasation in these regions represents a source of extraarticular pain not accounted for by the above neuroanatomy, and not necessarily amenable to the existing locoregional analgesic options.

REGIONAL ANESTHESIA TECHNIQUES
Lumbar Plexus Block

The lumbar plexus gives rise to many of the sensory nerves relevant to analgesia in hip arthroscopy. The LFCN innervates most of the cutaneous portal sites, and the FN, ON, and AON innervate the anterior capsule and bony structures. Today a lumbar plexus

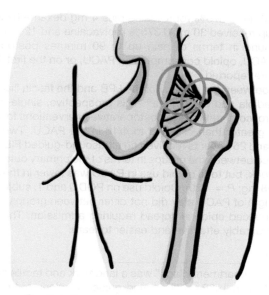

○ Sciatic nerve
○ Superior gluteal nerve
○ Nerve to quadratus femoris +
    Inferior gluteal nerve

Fig. 3. Innervation of the posterior hip joint. Colored circles represent portions of the capsule and joint innervated by the sciatic nerve (*green*), superior gluteal nerve (*pink*), and the nerve to the quadratus femoris and inferior gluteal nerve (*orange*).

block (LPB) refers to a posterior approach where the needle is passed between lumbar transverse processes into the psoas major. This was initially described by Chayen and colleagues[20] in 1976 as a "psoas compartment block" and has been technically refined over the years.[21] Because of the depth of the block, it is considered technically challenging and is associated with complications such as unintentional epidural or spinal injection,[22] and injury to retroperitoneal structures.

In a prospective single-blinded randomized control trial by YaDeau et al.,[23] 84 hip arthroscopy patients were randomized to either a preoperative LPB or control. Both groups received sedation before the study intervention, followed by operative anesthesia under combined spinal epidural. The control group patients were sedated and positioned for LPB, with no needle insertion, but identical bandage placement. Using generalized estimating equations modeling, a small but significant reduction was found in the LPB group for the primary outcome of pain at rest in the postanesthesia care unit (PACU; −0.9 points on a 10-point scale, $P = .037$). Mean pain scores at rest were 3.3 versus 4.2 in the control group ($P = .048$). However, there was no significant difference in PACU analgesic usage, PACU pain with movement, patient satisfaction, or postdischarge pain. The LPB group had several complications, with 2 patients falling in the hospital bathroom without injury and 1 patient admitted for epidural spread and subsequent urinary retention. Two control group patients were admitted: one for oxygen desaturation and one for intractable pain and nausea.

In a single-blinded study, Scanaliato and colleagues[24] randomized patients to preoperative LPB versus intraoperative pericapsular injection. The 32 patients in the LPB group received 40 mL 0.375% ropivacaine plus 4 mg dexamethasone, whereas the pericapsular group received 30 mL 0.375% ropivacaine and 12 mg morphine. No differences were found in terms of pain up to 90 minutes postoperatively, time to discharge from PACU, opioid consumption in PACU, or on the first 2 PODs. No major complications were reported.

A comparison between the efficacy of the LPB and the fascia iliaca block (FIB) was conducted by Badiola and colleagues[25] This prospective, single-blinded study randomized hip arthroscopy patients to postoperative interventions for patients expressing a pain score greater than or equal to 4/10 in the PACU. Twenty-three patients received an LPB and 25 patients received an ultrasound-guided FIB. The investigators found no difference between the groups in terms of the primary outcome of pain 15 minutes after the block, but total opioid use in PACU was lower in the LPB group (mean 20.80 mg vs 16.98 mg; $P = .020$). Opioid use on POD 0 and 1, subjective quality of the recovery, and length of PACU stay did not differ between groups. One patient in the LPB group experienced epidural spread requiring admission. The group concluded that FIB was comparably effective and easier to learn.

Fascia Iliaca Block

The "fascia iliaca compartment block" was a landmark and tactile approach originally described by Dalens in 1989.[26] Ultrasound-guided versions of the block have since emerged culminating in a suprainguinal version by Hebbard.[27] All versions of the block share the same premise: injection of local anesthetic beneath the fascia iliaca in an attempt to block the FN, ON, and LFCN. Studies vary in terms of which approach is used, an important distinction because ultrasound-guided suprainguinal versions are more successful in reaching the higher lumbar plexus branches innervating the hip.[28]

Behrends and colleagues conducted a prospective double-blinded trial in which hip arthroscopy patients were randomized to receive either preoperative ultrasound-guided suprainguinal (FIB) or saline placebo injection.[29] Thirty-eight patients received the suprainguinal FIB and 40 patients received a placebo injection at the same site. All patients received intraarticular (IA) injection of 10-mL ropivacaine 0.2% at procedure end. There was no difference in pain or opioid use in the block group compared to the placebo group in the recovery room or within the first 24 hours at home. There was also no difference in postoperative nausea and vomiting (PONV), walking ability, or patient satisfaction. However, the group did find a significant decrease in quadriceps strength in the FIB group as measured by a stationary dynamometer 30 minutes after the procedure, and a greater number of falls in the treatment group (4 vs 1, relative risk: 4.1; 95% confidence interval, 0.5–35.0). The investigators felt that a preoperative FIB is not effective due in part to incomplete coverage of the joint, and criticized the potential fall risk. They further speculated that the reason previous studies utilizing postoperative blocks showed a treatment effect had to do with patient selection, placebo effect, ability to perceive decreased nociception in the setting of incomplete coverage, and adaptive or stress-induced analgesia (pain is perceived to be less when preceded by a more painful stimulus).

A similarly designed study was performed by Huang and colleagues,[30] using an ultrasound-guided FIB below the inguinal ligament. In this prospective, single-blinded trial, 27 patients undergoing hip arthroscopy received a preoperative FIB and 33 received no preoperative intervention. Patients were randomized according to the day they had surgery, with all patients on a single day assigned to a single intervention. Surgeons and anesthesiologists were blinded to the randomization scheme. Patients remained unblinded. There were no differences between groups in terms of postoperative pain in PACU or on PODs 1, 2, 4, and 7. There were no differences in morphine equivalent dose, or patient satisfaction with pain control from operative day through POD 7.

Garner and colleagues' 2017 prospective single-blinded randomized study found relative ineffectiveness of FIB compared with local anesthetic infiltration (LAI).[31] Although the block technique is poorly described, the reader can infer that the FIB was likely infrainguinal and performed with ultrasound guidance. Patients were randomized to a preoperative ultrasound-guided FIB after induction of anesthesia (26 patients) versus LAI of the portal tracts at the end of the procedure (20 patients) using the same local anesthetic solution. The study was terminated early after it was found that the FIB group had significantly greater pain at 1-h postoperatively than the LAI group (mean 3.4/10 vs 5.5/10, P = .02) and required significantly higher doses of opioids and other analgesics within the first hour postoperatively (mean intravenous [IV] morphine 2.4 LAI vs 5.5 FICB, P = .050). There was no significant difference in pain between the 2 groups at 6 and 24 hours, nor was there a difference in 24-h opioid consumption. The FIB group had a greater incidence of nausea and vomiting at 6 and 24 hours although no statistical measurement was offered. The authors theorized that the LAI may have diffused beyond the capsule, anesthetizing the sciatic and gluteal branches that the FIB failed to block. They also offered that arthroscopic fluid could potentially wash away the local anesthetic from the preoperative FIB.

A randomized control trial by Glomset and colleagues[32] compared preoperative ultrasound-guided suprainguinal FIB with IA injection in an unblinded fashion. A total of 41 patients were enrolled in the FIB arm, and 43 in the IA arm. Injectates differed in terms of the types of local anesthetics, concentrations, volumes, and adjuvants both between and within study groups. The investigators found no significant differences in terms of pain scores at multiple time points in the PACU, and at 2, 6, and 12 weeks postoperatively. There was no significant difference between groups in terms of opioid use, PONV, or PACU recovery time, and neither group had complications.

FN Block

An FNB involves the injection of local anesthetic circumferentially around the FN, lateral to the femoral artery, and under the fascia iliaca. Modern methods may in some ways be mechanistically similar to infrainguinal fascia iliaca approaches because a local anesthetic is deposited in the same subfascial compartment in both approaches. With an FNB, the distance from the LFCN is greater and the local anesthetic volume requirement is lower. Interestingly, the few randomized control trials evaluating FNB for hip arthroscopy found it to be effective for pain control, in contrast to FIB.

Xing and colleagues' 2015 triple-blinded randomized control trial examined the ability of a preoperative FNB to control pain in hip arthroscopy patients.[33] A total of 27 patients received a preoperative ultrasound-guided FNB with 20 mL of 0.5% bupivacaine and 23 received a saline placebo block. Opioid consumption was significantly lower in the FNB group at 48 hours (mean 10.9 ± 12.5 vs 26.6 ± 24.6, P = .006), though not at 24 hours or 7 days postoperatively. Postoperative pain scores were significantly less in the FNB group at 30 minutes, and 1, 2, 4, and 6 hours postoperatively. No pain differences were found at 24 and 48 hours postoperatively. The FNB group had significantly more falls than the control group (6 of 27 vs 0 of 23, P = .025) leading the authors to recommend against routine use.

Ward and colleagues[34] studied the effects of a postoperative FNB compared to IV morphine. If pain score was 7 or greater in PACU, patients were randomized to either ultrasound and nerve stimulator-guided FNB versus IV morphine for pain control. The authors did not perform a power analysis, performed no blinding, did not record pain scores or opioid consumption, and made little mention of how additional analgesia was offered in the treatment group. Outcome measures were PACU duration, incidence of nausea and vomiting, and patient satisfaction with pain control on POD 1. A total of 20 patients received FNB and 16 patients received both IV and oral narcotics. FNB patients were significantly more likely to be satisfied with postoperative pain control than the IV narcotic group (90% vs 25%, P < .0001), had a shorter time to discharge from PACU than the IV narcotic group (177.85 ± 17.34 minutes vs 216.00 ± 19.48 minutes, P < .0001) and had a much lower incidence of PONV (10% vs 75% in the IV narcotics group, P < 0.001).

SURGICAL INFILTRATION AND IA INJECTION TECHNIQUES

The prospective double-blind randomized control trial by Shlaifer and colleagues[35] found greater pain control with periacetabular (PA) as compared with IA injection for hip arthroscopy. A total of 21 patients received a preoperative IA injection and 21 patients received a preoperative PA injection, both using 20 mL of bupivacaine 0.5%. Visual analog scale (VAS) scores were significantly lower at 30 minutes and 18 hours postoperatively in the PA group (0.667 ± 1.49 vs 2.11 ± 2.29; P < .045 and 2.62 ± 2.2 vs 4.79 ± 2.6; P < .009), though there were no differences between groups in VAS scores at 1, 2, 6, or 12 hours. Length of stay in the postoperative analgesia recovery room was significantly less for the PA group (2:03 vs 03:33, P = .007). There were no differences in the groups in terms of analgesic consumption.

In Philippi and colleagues' single-blinded trial,[36] patients undergoing hip arthroscopy were randomized to receive extracapsular LAI with 20 mL of 0.25% bupivacaine-epinephrine (1:200,000) or no LAI just before closure. A total of 36 patients received LAI and 37 received no LAI. There was a significant decrease in PACU VAS scores for the LAI group (mean 6.16 vs 7.35, P = .009), but no significant difference in discharge PACU pain scores. The groups had no differences in terms of length of stay in PACU (median 97 minutes vs 118 minutes, P = .09) or opioid consumption (10 MME vs 14 MME, P = .09).

Baker and colleagues[37] performed a double-blinded randomized trial wherein 73 patients undergoing hip arthroscopy received 10 mL of 0.25% bupivacaine either IA or around portal sites. 40 patients received IA injection and 33 received portal site injections. There was no difference in VAS scores between groups until 6 hours postoperatively when the portal site group had significantly lower scores (P = .0036), but also required significantly more rescue analgesia immediately after surgery (2.33 mg vs 0.57 mg, P = .036). Morgenthaler and colleagues found stronger support for IA injection in their 2007 double-blinded randomized control trial.[38] A total of 13 patients received 20 mL of 0.25% bupivacaine IA at the end of surgery and 13 patients received 0.9% saline IA. Postoperatively, the group that received IA bupivacaine had significantly lower VAS scores at rest (mean 17.5 vs 27.5 using the 100-point scale, P = .05) and during movement (mean 23 vs 46, P = .001).

NEW TECHNIQUES: ULTRASOUND-GUIDED FASCIAL PLANE BLOCKS
Pericapsular Nerve Group Block

With advancements in ultrasound technology facilitating better visualization and understanding of anatomy, there has been increased interest in targeting local anesthetic injection to tissue planes and compartments, with the goal of anesthetizing smaller distal sensory nerve branches with less risk of motor blockade. One recent example is the pericapsular nerve group block or PENG block, nicknamed for one of its creators

Philip Peng.[39] The block capitalizes on anatomic studies of the anterior hip innervation mentioned previously,[10] by injecting local anesthetic in the plane between the iliopsoas tendon and the illiopubic eminence, where articular branches of the FN, ON, and AON may travel (**Fig. 4**). In many ways, this technique more resembles surgical LAI than traditional peripheral nerve blocks. This novel technique has not yet been evaluated in a clinical trial for hip arthroscopy, but recent evidence does support its effectiveness as a motor-sparing analgesic method for hip fractures.

A 2021 double-blinded comparative trial conducted by Lin and colleagues[40] randomized 60 patients undergoing hip fracture to receive either a preoperative FNB or PENG block. The group receiving the PENG block experienced less pain (63% experiencing no pain, 27% mild pain, and 10% moderate to severe pain vs 30%, 27%, and 36% in the FNB group, respectively, $P = .04$). The PENG block group also had better preserved PACU and POD 1 quadriceps strength as assessed by Oxford muscle strength grading (60% intact vs 0% intact, $P < .001$). There were no differences between groups in terms of opiate use, complications, or length of hospital stay.

Sahoo and colleagues[41] conducted a prospective cohort study in which 20 patients with hip fractures (18 femoral neck and 2 intertrochanteric) received PENG blocks before surgery. Pain significantly decreased after PENG block. The initial mean pain score at rest 7.45/10 fell to 0.75/10, and initial mean pain while moving 9.45/10 decreased to 1.34/10 after the intervention ($P < .001$).

Allard and colleagues retrospectively reviewed outcomes of patients undergoing femoral neck repair that received a preoperative PENG block versus an FNB.[42] No differences were identified in terms of postoperative opioid consumption, pain intensity, time to ambulation, incidence of opioid-related side effects, or length of hospital stay. However, postoperative muscle strength was preserved in the PENG block group compared with the FNB group as measured by the Medical Research Council's immediate postoperative mobility scale (5/5 vs 2/5, $P = .001$).

Quadratus Lumborum Block

The quadratus lumborum (QL) muscle is seated between layers of the thoracolumbar fascia (TLF), abutting the psoas major anteromedially, the abdominal wall muscles laterally, and the latissimus dorsi and erector spinae muscles posteriorly. Injection in various locations around the QL has been used for abdominal wall analgesia; however, there is interest in its use for hip analgesia as there may be communication between

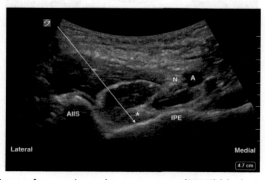

Fig. 4. Ultrasound image for a pericapsular nerve group (PENG) block. Needle (*arrow*) passes from lateral to medial until the tip is between the iliopsoas tendon (*) and the iliopubic eminence below. A, femoral artery; AIIS, anterior inferior iliac spine; IPE, iliopubic eminence; N, femoral nerve.

layers of the TLF with nerves of the lumbar plexus and paravertebral space[43,44] (**Fig. 5**). Given the novel indication, there are no studies related to hip arthroscopy; however, we present evidence for its effectiveness in hip arthroplasty. Several approaches exist, with the transmuscular or anterior version showing greater promise. Here the local is deposited between the QL and psoas muscles.

He and colleagues' 2020 double-blinded randomized control trial found that preoperative anterior/transmuscular QLB was an effective means of pain control for total hip arthroplasty.[45] A total of 41 patients received a QLB, whereas 42 patients received a saline placebo block. The QLB group experienced less postoperative pain at rest at 6, 12, 24, 36, and 48 hours postoperatively ($P < .001$) and during movement at 24, 36, and 48 hours ($P < .001$). Morphine use in the QLB group was significantly lower than the control group during POD 1 (mean 16 vs 34 mg, $P < .001$) and on POD 2 (mean 13 vs 17.4, $P < .001$). Incidence of nausea (3 vs 13 participants, $P = .006$) and vomiting (3 vs 11 participants, $P = .022$) were significantly more common in the control group.

Brixel and colleagues conducted a double-blinded clinical trial in which patients undergoing total hip arthroplasty were randomized to preoperatively receive a posterior QLB with either 0.33% ropivacaine or normal saline.[46] In the posterior approach, the local is injected behind the QL and anterior to the latissimus. A total of 50 patients received ropivacaine and 50 patients received the control block. There was no significant difference between groups in any measure, including 24-h total morphine consumption, pain scores at extubation, 2, 6, 12, and 24 hours postoperatively, intraoperative opioid consumption, motor blockade, times to first standing, time to ambulation, hospital length of stay, or adverse events.

In Aoyama's 2020 unblinded randomized control trial, continuous anterior/transmuscular QLB was compared with continuous FNB for total hip arthroplasty.[47] A total of 13 patients received the QLB and 11 received the FNB interventions, both with catheters. After surgery, all patients received a continuous infusion of 0.125% levobupivacaine at 4 mL/h via the catheter. VAS scores out of 100 on movement were significantly less in the FNB group at 6 hours (mean 67 vs 38; $P = .008$) and 24 hours (mean 60 vs 39; $P = .018$), but there was no difference at 12 and 48 hours. There were no differences between groups in terms of VAS scores at rest, at 6, 12, 24, or 48 hours postoperatively, as well as in patient-controlled analgesia (PCA) demands, rescue

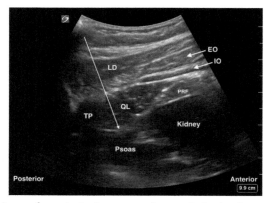

Fig. 5. Ultrasound image for anterior/transmuscular quadratus lumborum block. The needle path (*long white arrow*) is anteromedial, past the lumbar transverse process (TP), through the QL until it reaches the anterior thoracolumbar fascia separating the QL from the psoas. EO, external oblique; IO, internal oblique; LD, latissimus dorsi; PRF, perirenal fat.

analgesic use, or complications. Sensory evaluations showed a more inconsistent pattern in the QLB group, with 6/10 showing no discernible cutaneous blockade at 6 hours (P = .006). In subgroup analysis, those that did have sensory block had less pain. The authors speculated that block execution and local anesthetic spread may be affected by age, habitus, and mobility.

SUMMARY

Pain associated with hip arthroscopy may be severe,[2] and many locoregional techniques have been used in an attempt to provide opioid-sparing analgesia. Regional nerve blocks such as femoral, fascia iliaca, and lumbar plexus have had some mixed successes. Some studies do show a reduction in pain and analgesic consumption, but at the expense of motor weakness, falls, and in the case of lumbar plexus blockade, more serious complications like epidural spread or retroperitoneal injuries.[22] The sensory innervation of the hip is complex, and to date, most regional techniques only target the anterior joint nerves. Although this logically should reduce pain to some extent, there are reasons why certain preoperative blocks may not be successful: extravasated arthroscopic fluid diluting the local anesthetic[31] and difficulty perceiving appreciable analgesia in the setting of residual pain from other unblocked nociceptive regions.[29] LAI may reduce pain, and when performed thoughtfully, should avoid weakness. Periacetabular injection seems to be better than IA injection, which makes good sense methodologically. The PENG block places local anesthetic above the acetabulum on the iliopubic eminence, using a similar neuroanatomic basis, and is attractive for its lack of associated motor weakness. Quadratus lumborum blocks also show promise in the setting of other hip procedures, and these 2 new ultrasound-guided approaches deserve formal clinical evaluation for hip arthroscopy. Greater attention could also be paid to the posterior joint and extraarticular sources of pain. More thoughtful anatomic infiltration, either intraoperative or through the use of ultrasound, may be the key to optimal analgesia without ambulatory impairment.

CLINICS CARE POINTS

- Fascia iliaca blocks performed preoperatively have not been shown to reduce pain or opioid consumption when compared to placebo, local anesthetic infiltration, or intraarticular injection.
- They are additionally associated with quadriceps weakness,Femoral nerve blocks performed preoperatively have been shown to reduce pain scores and opioid consumption, but are associated with an increased number of falls.
- Periacetabular injection of local anesthetic may be superior to intraarticular injection with respect to postoperative pain scores and recovery room length of stay.
- In cohort studies, pericapsular nerve group block reduces pain associated with hip fractures, while preserving muscle function.
- Anterior quadratus lumborum blocks have been proven to reduce pain and opioid consumption for total hip arthroplasty.

DISCLOSURE

Dr F.W. Gwathmey is a consultant and speaker for Arthrex, a consultant for Allosource, and receives royalties from Elsevier. None of the other authors have any disclosures with regard to this article.

REFERENCES

1. Anciano Granadillo V, Cancienne JM, Gwathmey FW, et al. Trends, risk factors for prolonged use, and complications. Arthrosc - J Arthroscopic Relat Surg 2018; 34(8):2359–67.

2. Baker JF, Byrne DP, Hunter K, et al. Post-operative opiate requirements after hip arthroscopy. Knee Surg Sports Traumatol Arthrosc 2011;(8):19. https://doi.org/10.1007/s00167-010-1248-4.

3. Ramos L, Kraeutler MJ, Marty E, et al. Tolerance in the early postoperative period after hip arthroscopy. Orthopaedic J Sports Med 2020;(10):8. https://doi.org/10.1177/2325967120960689.

4. Sivasundaram L, Trivedi NN, Kim CY, et al. Emergency department utilization after elective hip arthroscopy. Arthrosc - J Arthroscopic Relat Surg 2020;36(6): 1575–83.e1.

5. Nielsen KC, Steele SM. Outcome after regional anaesthesia in the ambulatory setting – is it really worth it? Best Pract Res Clin Anaesthesiol 2002;(2):16. https://doi.org/10.1053/bean.2002.0244.

6. Byrd JWT, Pappas JN, Pedley MJ. Hip arthroscopy: an anatomic study of portal placement and relationship to the extra-articular structures. Arthroscopy 1995;(4):11. https://doi.org/10.1016/0749-8063(95)90193-0.

7. Tamura S, Nishii T, Takao M, et al. Differences in the locations and modes of labral tearing between dysplastic hips and those with femoroacetabular impingement. Bone Joint J 2013;1320–5, 95-B(10).

8. Birnbaum K, Prescher A, Heßler S, et al. The sensory innervation of the hip joint - an anatomical study. Surg Radiologic Anat 1997;19(6):371–5.

9. Simons M, Amin N, Cushner F, et al. Characterization of the neural anatomy in the hip joint to optimize periarticular regional anesthesia in total hip arthroplasty. J Surg Orthopaedic Adv 2015;(04):24. https://doi.org/10.3113/JSOA, 2015.0221.

10. Short AJ, Barnett JJG, Gofeld M, et al. Anatomic study of innervation of the anterior hip capsule: implication for image-guided intervention. Reg Anesth Pain Med 2018;43(2):186–92.

11. Laumonerie P, Dalmas Y, Tibbo ME, et al. Sensory innervation of the hip joint and referredpain: a systematic review of the literature. Pain Med 2021;22(5):1149–57.

12. Tomlinson J, Zwirner J, Ondruschka B, et al. Innervation of the hip joint capsular complex: A systematic review of histological and immunohistochemical studies and their clinical implications for contemporary treatment strategies in total hip arthroplasty. PLoS ONE 2020;(2):15. https://doi.org/10.1371/journal.pone.0229128.

13. Alzaharani A, Bali K, Gudena R, et al. The innervation of the human acetabular labrum and hip joint: An anatomic study. BMC Musculoskelet Disord 2014;(1): 15. https://doi.org/10.1186/1471-2474-15-41.

14. Gerhardt M, Johnson K, Atkinson R, et al. Characterisation and classification of the neural anatomy in the human hip joint. HIP Int 2012;(1):22. https://doi.org/10.5301/HIP, 2012.9042.

15. Haversath M, Hanke J, Landgraeber S, et al. The distribution of nociceptive innervation in the painful hip. Bone Joint J 2013. https://doi.org/10.1302/0301-620X.95B6.30262. 95-B(6).

16. Kampa RJ, Prasthofer A, Lawrence-Watt DJ, et al. The internervous safe zone for incision of the capsule of the hip A CADAVER STUDY. J Bone Joint Surg Br 2007; 89(7). https://doi.org/10.1302/0301-620X.89B7.

17. Tan CO, Chong YM, Tran P, et al. Surgical predictors of acute postoperative pain after hip arthroscopy. BMC Anesthesiol 2015;(1):15. https://doi.org/10.1186/s12871-015-0077-x.

18. Hinzpeter J, Barrientos C, Barahona M, et al. Fluid extravasation related to hip arthroscopy: a prospective computed tomography–based study. Orthopaedic J Sports Med 2015;3(3). https://doi.org/10.1177/2325967115573222.

19. Haskins SC, Desai NA, Fields KG, et al. Diagnosis of intraabdominal fluid extravasation after hip arthroscopy with point-of-care ultrasonography can identify patients at an increased risk for postoperative pain. Anesth Analg 2017;(3):124. https://doi.org/10.1213/ANE.0000000000001435.

20. Chayen D, Nathan H, Chayen M. The psoas compartment block. Anesthesiology 1976;45(1):95–9.

21. Capdevila X, Macaire P, Dadure C, et al. Continuous psoas compartment block for postoperative analgesia after total hip arthroplasty: new landmarks, technical guidelines, and clinical evaluation. Anesth Analg 2002;94. Available at: https://journals.lww.com/anesthesia-analgesia.

22. Macaire P, Gaertner E, Choquet O. Le Bloc du plexus lombaire est-il dangereux?. In: Sfar, editor. Evaluation et Traitement de La Douleur. 2nd edition. Elsevier et SFAR; 2002. p. 37–50, 200.

23. YaDeau JT, Tedore T, Goytizolo EA, et al. Lumbar plexus blockade reduces pain after hip arthroscopy: a prospective randomized controlled trial. Anesth Analg 2012;(4):115.

24. Scanaliato JP, Christensen D, Polmear MM, et al. Prospective single-blinded randomized controlled trial comparing pericapsular injection versus lumbar plexus peripheral nerve block for hip arthroscopy. Am J Sports Med 2020;48(11):2740–6.

25. Badiola I, Liu J, Huang S, et al. A comparison of the fascia iliaca block to the lumbar plexus block in providing analgesia following arthroscopic hip surgery: A randomized controlled clinical trial. J Clin Anesth 2018;49:26–9. https://doi.org/10.1016/j.jclinane.2018.05.012. Available at:.

26. Dalens B, Vanneuville G, Tanguy A. Comparison of the fascia iliaca compartment block with the 3-in-1 block in children. Anesth Analg 1989;69(6):705–13. Available at: http://www.ncbi.nlm.nih.gov/pubmed/2589650.

27. Hebbard P, Ivanusic J, Sha S. Ultrasound-guided supra-inguinal fascia iliaca block: a cadaveric evaluation of a novel approach. Anaesthesia 2011;(4):66. https://doi.org/10.1111/j.1365-2044.2011.06628.x.

28. Vermeylen K, Desmet M, Leunen I, et al. Supra-inguinal injection for fascia iliaca compartment block results in more consistent spread towards the lumbar plexus than an infra-inguinal injection: a volunteer study. Reg Anesth Pain Med 2019;(4):44. https://doi.org/10.1136/rapm-2018-100092.

29. Behrends M, Yap EN, Zhang AL, et al. Preoperative fascia iliaca block does not improve analgesia after arthroscopic hip surgery, but causes quadriceps muscles weakness: a randomized, double-blind trial. Anesthesiology 2018;129(3):536–43.

30. Huang M, Wages J, Henry A, et al. Should preoperative fascia iliaca block be used for hip arthroscopic labral repair and femoroacetabular impingement treatment? a prospective single blinded randomized study. Arthroscopy 2020;36(4):1039–44.

31. Garner M, Alshameeri Z, Sardesai A, et al. A prospective randomized controlled trial comparing the efficacy of fascia iliaca compartment block versus local anesthetic infiltration after hip arthroscopic surgery. Arthroscopy 2017;33(1):125–32.

32. Glomset JL, Kim E, Tokish JM, et al. Reduction of postoperative hip arthroscopy pain with an ultrasound-guided fascia iliaca block: a prospective randomized controlled trial. Am J Sports Med 2020;48(3):682–8.
33. Xing JG, Abdallah FW, Brull R, et al. Preoperative femoral nerve block for hip arthroscopy: a randomized, triple-masked controlled trial. Am J Sports Med 2015;43(11):2680–7.
34. Ward JP, Albert DB, Altman R, et al. Are femoral nerve blocks effective for early postoperative pain management after hip arthroscopy? Arthroscopy 2012;28(8): 1064–9. https://doi.org/10.1016/j.arthro.2012.01.003. Available at:.
35. Shlaifer A, Sharfman ZT, Martin HD, et al. Preemptive analgesia in hip arthroscopy: a randomized controlled trial of preemptive periacetabular or intra-articular bupivacaine in addition to postoperative intra-articular bupivacaine. Arthrosc The J Arthroscopic Relat Surg 2017;33(1):118–24.
36. Philippi MT, Kahn TL, Adeyemi TF, et al. Extracapsular local infiltration analgesia in hip arthroscopy patients: a randomized, prospective study. J hip preservation Surg 2018;5(3):226–32.
37. Baker JF, Mcguire CM, Byrne DP, et al. Analgesic control after hip arthroscopy: a randomised, double-blinded trial comparing portal with intra-articular infiltration of bupivacaine. HIP Int 2011;21(3):373–7.
38. Morgenthaler K, Bauer C, Ziegeler S, et al. Intraartikuläre Bupivacaingabe bei Hüftgelenkarthroskopie. Der Anaesthesist 2007;56(11):1128–32.
39. Girón-Arango L, Peng PWH, Chin KJ, et al. Pericapsular nerve group (peng) block for hip fracture. Reg Anesth Pain Med 2018. https://doi.org/10.1097/AAP. 0000000000000847.
40. Lin D-Y, Morrison C, Brown B, et al. Pericapsular nerve group (PENG) block provides improved short-term analgesia compared with the femoral nerve block in hip fracture surgery: a single-center double-blinded randomized comparative trial. Reg Anesth & Pain Med 2021;46(5):398.
41. Sahoo RK, Jadon A, Sharma SK, et al. Peri-capsular nerve group block provides excellent analgesia in hip fractures and positioning for spinal anaesthesia: a prospective cohort study. Indian J Anaesth 2020;64(10):898–900.
42. Allard C, Pardo E, de la Jonquière C, et al. Comparison between femoral block and PENG block in femoral neck fractures: A cohort study. PloS one 2021; 16(6):e0252716.
43. Carline L, McLeod GA, Lamb C. A cadaver study comparing spread of dye and nerve involvement after three different quadratus lumborum blocks. Br J Anaesth 2016;(3):117. https://doi.org/10.1093/bja/aew224.
44. Dam M, Moriggl B, Hansen CK, et al. The pathway of injectate spread with the transmuscular quadratus lumborum block: a cadaver study. Anesth Analg 2017;(1):125. https://doi.org/10.1213/ANE.0000000000001922.
45. He J, Zhang L, He WY, et al. Ultrasound-guided transmuscular quadratus lumborum block reduces postoperative pain intensity in patients undergoing total hip arthroplasty: a randomized, double-blind, placebo-controlled trial. Pain Res Manag 2020;2020:1035182. https://doi.org/10.1155/2020/1035182.
46. Brixel SM, Biboulet P, Swisser F, et al. Posterior quadratus lumborum block in total hip arthroplasty: a randomized controlled trial. Anesthesiology 2021;134(5): 722–33.
47. Aoyama Y, Sakura S, Abe S, et al. Continuous quadratus lumborum block and femoral nerve block for total hip arthroplasty: a randomized study. J Anesth 2020;34(3):413–20.

Anesthesia for the Patient Undergoing Knee Procedures

Grant Neely, MD*, Nicole Hollis, MD, Cy Mozingo, MD

KEYWORDS

- Anesthesia • Knee surgery • Nerve block • Regional anesthesia

KEY POINTS

- The primary approach to anesthesia for most patients undergoing knee procedures is general anesthesia or spinal anesthesia with multimodal analgesic modalities, including oral and intravenous medications along with supplemental regional anesthetic techniques.
- Innervation to the knee joint is complex with contributions from the femoral, sciatic, and obturator nerves and their articular branches.
- Regional anesthesia blocks provide broad analgesic coverage to the knee, ranging from complete anesthesia during surgery to motor-sparing analgesic coverage.
- Anesthetic and analgesic options for knee surgery depend primarily on the type and acuity of the procedure being performed, individual patient characteristics, and anesthetic and surgical goals.

INTRODUCTION

Hundreds of thousands of knee-related procedures and surgeries occur every year in the United States. According to the Agency for Healthcare Research and Quality, more than 754,000 knee replacements alone were performed in 2017.[1] These procedures occur in a myriad of different surgical settings, including large academic centers, private hospitals, and outpatient surgery centers. As these procedures are performed on a wide range of patients with variability in age, comorbidities, and specific pathology requiring surgery, anesthesia for patients undergoing knee procedures requires proper patient selection and optimization for the type of anesthetic delivered.

As mentioned earlier, anesthetic techniques may vary depending on patient and surgical-related factors. Also important are the chronicity and severity of the injury itself. Additional considerations are required for patients suffering traumatic or acute

West Virginia University Department of Anesthesiology, 1 Medical Center Drive, PO Box 8255, Morgantown, WV 26508, USA
* Corresponding author.
E-mail address: neelyg@hsc.wvu.edu

Clin Sports Med 41 (2022) 247–261
https://doi.org/10.1016/j.csm.2021.11.002
0278-5919/22/© 2021 Elsevier Inc. All rights reserved.

injuries in comparison with those with subacute or chronic pathology. Considerations may include risk for compartment syndrome, degree of analgesia required after surgery, and requirement for ambulation and use of the operative leg during rehabilitation. Therefore, detailed knowledge of the anatomy and innervation of the lower extremity is required to understand regional anesthetic approaches to analgesia as well as the location and severity of pain to be expected after each type of surgery. Simplified, most of the dermatome, myotome, and osteotome innervation of the knee is supplied by the femoral nerve with direct or articular branches from the sciatic and obturator nerves to the posterior and medial aspects of the knee joint, respectively.[2]

Regional nerve blocks play an important role in a multimodal analgesic approach to patients undergoing knee surgeries. A variety of blocks can be performed with each nerve block offering a different degree and location of analgesic coverage to the knee joint. Regional procedures can contribute to complete analgesia and anesthesia to the knee or can be used in concert with a spinal or general anesthetic technique to provide postoperative analgesia. An adductor canal block, for example, may provide postoperative analgesia with a clinically motor-sparing effect, allowing for early ambulation if indicated.[2] Nerve blocks may be performed before or after the planned procedure, and special consideration of the risks, benefits, complications, and alternatives of regional anesthesia should be addressed based on the type of surgery and specific patient characteristics. For example, in the professional athlete undergoing knee surgery, effective communication must occur between the anesthesiologist, surgeon, and patient so that all involved understand the risks and benefits of an elective regional nerve block.[3]

Regardless of the utilization of regional nerve blocks, all patients undergoing surgery for knee-related injuries benefit from a multidisciplinary approach utilizing thoughtful patient selection, preoperative optimization, a balanced anesthetic with multimodal analgesia, and proper early postoperative mobilization and oral intake. Multimodal analgesia improves pain control, decreases postoperative care unit time, and reduces overall opioid consumption. In addition to regional anesthesia, opioid-sparing analgesic regimens typically include acetaminophen, gabapentanoids, NMDA antagonists, and nonsteroidal anti-inflammatory agents when clinically appropriate.[4] Multimodal analgesia is a vital component of a balanced anesthetic for both acute, subacute, and chronic knee injuries requiring surgery.

DISCUSSION
Acute Knee Injuries

Acute traumatic injuries to the lower extremities can benefit from regional anesthetic techniques for pain control. However, regional anesthetics may interfere with postoperative neurovascular evaluations and the risks and benefits should be considered. After an acute sports-related injury requiring surgical intervention, avoidance of regional anesthetic techniques may seem prudent to properly evaluate for sensory or motor dysfunction. For example, in the case of an inside-out lateral meniscal repair or a multiligament repair with a posterolateral corner injury, one might consider offering a postoperative sciatic nerve block only after sensory and motor function were evaluated after the procedure.

Neurologic injury is a potential rare complication after a peripheral nerve block. Preexisting nerve injury secondary to trauma is a relative contraindication for a peripheral nerve block due to concern of worsening the nerve injury.[5-7]

Compartment syndrome occurs with excessive pressure within muscle compartments, and the potential for ischemia and muscle necrosis. High-risk categories for compartment syndrome include tibial plateau fractures, crush injuries, and prolonged extrication.[8] Left untreated, compartment syndrome can result in severe ischemia resulting in amputation, renal failure from rhabdomyolysis, and cardiac arrhythmias. Pain is classically considered a cardinal sign in the diagnosis of compartment syndrome, and regional anesthesia techniques that provide dense analgesia have been thought to delay diagnosis and treatment. However, data suggest that regional anesthesia may not mask diagnosis and may, in fact, aid in its detection.[9] Therefore, the use of regional anesthesia in patients at high risk for compartment syndrome remains controversial. When regional anesthesia is planned for analgesic relief in patients at risk of compartment syndrome, dilute local anesthetic concentrations can be used to provide analgesia, avoid motor and dense sensory blockade, and allow for adequate physical assessment.[10]

Subacute and Chronic Knee Injuries

Subacute and chronic knee injuries requiring surgical intervention share the benefit of allowing for more time to perform proper patient selection for the surgical location in addition to optimization of comorbidities for the upcoming procedure. Given the complex innervation of the knee joint, general anesthesia is often the anesthetic of choice for most surgeries. However, most surgeries that can be performed under approximately 2 hours, such as total joint arthroplasty, should be completed successfully with a spinal anesthetic. Spinal anesthesia offers some benefits for total joint arthroplasty patients when compared with general anesthesia, including decreased length of stay, decreased surgical site injection, and decreased blood loss. The choice between general and spinal anesthesia depends on several factors, such as patient preference, likelihood of successful spinal placement in patients with lumbar spine pathology, concomitant medications interfering with the hematologic process, patient comorbidities (eg, respiratory or valvular cardiac disease), and length of surgery.[11,12]

Regardless of the anesthetic technique, a multimodal analgesic approach remains the mainstay of a balanced anesthetic. Regional anesthesia provides excellent opioid-sparing analgesia for these patients and can be performed before or after surgery depending on the surgical approach and need for neurologic assessment postoperatively. This requires excellent communication between the anesthesiologist, surgeon, and patient. For patients undergoing surgery for subacute injuries, including ligamentous repair (eg, ACL, PCL, MCL), meniscus surgery, or patellar fracture, general anesthesia is typically used along with multimodal analgesia. If regional anesthetic blocks are used in conjunction with these surgeries, "single-shot" blocks are often used. Single-shot blocks with long-acting local anesthetics and adjuncts last approximately 12 to 18 hours and provide analgesia for the immediate postoperative period. This approach allows the patient to begin a multimodal oral analgesic regimen before block dissipation and avoid playing "catch-up" with pain control. Patients undergoing larger surgeries for chronic knee pathology, such as patellofemoral syndrome, chondromalacia patellae, medial patellofemoral ligament syndrome, or procedures involving an osteochondral autograft transfer system, may benefit from longer-acting regional anesthetic techniques (eg, femoral and sciatic blocks) with catheter placement to provide analgesia for multiple days postoperatively. This technique may allow the patient to participate in physical therapy and improve the range of motion earlier in the recovery process.

Innervation of the Knee

Critical to providing analgesia for knee surgery is understanding the cutaneous innervation of the knee, as well as the innervation to the knee joint and capsule. Although the cutaneous innervation is well-described, the sensory innervation of the knee joint is complex and varies between individuals.

- The cutaneous innervation of the anteromedial aspect of the knee is supplied by the femoral nerve via the anterior cutaneous nerve of the thigh and the saphenous nerve.
- The common fibular nerve, a branch of the sciatic nerve, innervates the posterolateral aspect.
- The posterior cutaneous nerve of the thigh innervates much of the posterior portion of the skin overlying the knee.

There has been debate regarding the sensory innervation of the knee joint and capsule because of interindividual variability. Cadaveric anatomic and ultrasonographic studies have indicated that substantial innervation to the medial knee capsule and retinaculum are provided by the nerve to the vastus medialis, saphenous nerve, anterior branch of the obturator nerve, and articular branches of the sciatic nerve.[13] Articular branches of the sciatic nerve and nerve to the vastus lateralis provide innervation to the superolateral portion of the knee joint. The common peroneal nerve supplies the inferolateral aspect of the joint. Significant variation has been encountered in sensory innervation of the posterior capsule. One cadaveric study revealed that branches from the posterior division of the obturator and tibial nerves supplied the posterior division in all subjects.[14] Articular branches of the common peroneal nerve were also present in the posterior capsule in 53% of individuals, whereas branches of the sciatic nerve were present in 20%. This study indicates that the tibial nerve provides sensory innervation to the entire posterior capsule with overlap of the superomedial aspect provided by the posterior division of the obturator nerve. When present, the common peroneal nerve and articular branches of the sciatic nerve innervate the superolateral portion of the posterior capsule, along with the tibial nerve.[14] The innervation of the knee joint is summarized in **Table 1**.

Regional Nerve Blocks

Regional anesthesia can provide beneficial opioid-sparing analgesia for patients undergoing knee surgery. Anesthesiologists performing peripheral nerve blocks must follow the standards of care when performing these procedures including conducting a thorough timeout and ensuring proper patient positioning, equipment, skin preparation, and local anesthetic. Standard procedures are summarized in **Table 2**.

Comprehensive (Surgical) Blocks for the Knee

The use of comprehensive nerve blocks for various knee surgeries may be beneficial in patients with multiple medical comorbidities, placing them at high risk for general anesthesia. For these types of cases, regional anesthesia techniques can be used as the primary anesthetic. Dense surgical anesthesia may be accomplished by a combination of lumbar plexus and sciatic nerve blocks utilizing high concentrations of local anesthetic, such as 0.5% ropivacaine or bupivacaine. In addition, the individual nerve of the lumbar plexus (femoral, lateral femoral cutaneous, and obturator) can be blocked along with a sciatic nerve block.

Lumbar Plexus Block

The lumbar plexus is primarily formed from the L1-L4 spinal nerve roots. The nerve roots emerge from the vertebral foramen and run along the posterior portion of the psoas muscle. The major branches of the lumbar plexus include the femoral, lateral femoral cutaneous, and obturator nerves.

Table 1
Sensory innervation of the knee

Peripheral Nerve		Sensory Innervation	
	Branch	Cutaneous	Joint/Joint Capsule
Femoral	Saphenous	Anteromedial	Medial capsule and retinaculum
	Anterior cutaneous nerve of the thigh	Anteromedial	None
	Nerve to vastus medialis	None	Medial capsule and retinaculum
	Nerve to vastus lateralis	None	Superolateral capsule
Sciatic	Tibial	No cutaneous innervation at knee	Posterior and inferomedial capsule
	Common peroneal	Posterolateral	Inferolateral capsule, superolateral portion of posterior capsule
	Articular branches	None	Genicular branches to medial, superolateral, and posterior capsule
	Posterior cutaneous nerve of the thigh	Posterior	None
Obturator	Anterior branch	No cutaneous innervation at knee	Medial capsule and retinaculum
	Posterior branch	No cutaneous innervation at knee	Superomedial aspect of posterior capsule

- The femoral nerve supplies motor fibers to the quadriceps muscle and sensory fibers to the anteromedial thigh and medial aspect of the leg below the knee.
- The obturator nerve supplies motor branches to the adductor muscles of the hip and sensory to the medial thigh and knee joint.
- The lateral femoral cutaneous nerve provides sensory innervation to the antero-lateral thigh (**Fig. 1**).

The lumbar plexus block is the only technique that consistently blocks the femoral, lateral femoral cutaneous, and obturator nerves. Blocking the lumbar plexus can be completed by landmark or ultrasound guidance. Anesthesia to the knee may also be accomplished by individually blocking the nerve branches of the lumbar plexus more distally (**Fig. 2**).

Ultrasound-guided technique for lumbar plexus block

- The patient is positioned in the lateral decubitus position with the operative side up.
- The quadriceps muscle on the operative side should be easily visualized for twitch monitoring.
- At the level of the L4 transverse process, a low-frequency curvilinear ultrasound probe is placed in a transverse fashion to identify the L4 transverse process, psoas muscle, and lumbar plexus within the psoas muscle.
- The block needle is inserted in-plane lateral to the probe and directed medially.
- Patellar snap of the patellar tendon is the twitch that should be obtained.
- After correct needle positioning is confirmed, a lumbar plexus block is completed by injecting local anesthetic within the psoas muscle.

Table 2 Standard procedures for all peripheral nerve block procedures	
Timeout	Before sedation administration, confirm patient name, date of birth, and medical record number. Confirm surgical and anesthesia consents have been completed and correct surgery/block to be performed with corresponding correct sidedness. Review patient medication allergies, pertinent laboratories, and recent anticoagulation/antiplatelet therapy.
Position	Supine, lateral, or prone depending on block. Properly draped.
Equipment	Ultrasound machine with high-frequency linear probe (8–15 MHz) or low-frequency curvilinear probe (2–5 MHz) Supplemental oxygen if needed (nasal cannula, facemask) Emergency resuscitation equipment available
Syringe & Needle	20–30 mL syringes with 80–100 mm short-bevel nerve block needle
Skin Preparation	Chlorhexidine with alcohol
Local Anesthetic	Dependent on surgical indication and duration Short duration (2–6 h): mepivacaine 1.5% or lidocaine 1.5% Longer duration (12–18 h): bupivacaine or ropivacaine 0.2%–0.5%
Adjuvants	Minor prolongation of blockade. Each is associated with unique side effects. Dexamethasone (4 mg) Dexmedetomidine (1–2 μg/kg) Clonidine (25–50 μg) Epinephrine (2.5–5 μg/mL)

A lumbar plexus block is commonly used for perioperative analgesia. However, it can be used as a surgical anesthetic for hip or knee surgery when combined with a sciatic nerve block. Risks associated with a lumbar plexus block include bleeding, needle injury to viscera, and epidural spread.[15,16]

Sciatic Nerve Blocks

If complete anesthesia of the knee is desired for surgery using regional anesthesia, a sciatic nerve block must be performed. The sciatic nerve is formed via ventral rami of the L4-S3 nerve roots. As described previously, the sciatic nerve supplies cutaneous innervation to the posterior thigh, knee, and most of the lower leg, ankle, and foot. The

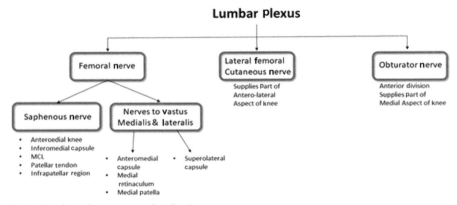

Fig. 1. Lumbar plexus nerve distribution.

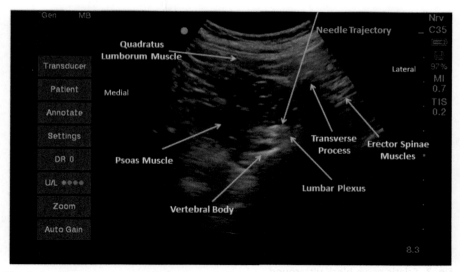

Fig. 2. Lumbar plexus nerve block ultrasound.

sciatic nerve also provides important articular branches to the knee capsule. The sciatic nerve can be blocked at various locations, both proximally and distally. Although proximal sciatic nerve blocks are frequently used along with the femoral block to provide analgesia in the posterior distribution for knee surgery, the sciatic block above the popliteal fossa also provides analgesic benefit for knee surgery.[17] Below, the subgluteal and popliteal approaches to the sciatic nerve block will be described, given their improved safety profiles and ultrasound visualization in comparison to the parasacral approach. The choice of local anesthetic is dependent on the surgical indication.

Proximal sciatic (subgluteal) approach
Ultrasound-guided technique to proximal sciatic nerve block
- With the patient in the lateral decubitus position, a low-frequency curvilinear probe is placed transversely over the posterior thigh.
- Once the femur is located, the probe is slid proximally to the greater trochanter.
- The probe is then transitioned medially from the greater trochanter to visualize the gluteus maximus in the center of the ultrasound image.
- At this location, the sciatic nerve lies deep to the gluteus maximus and superficial to the quadratus femoris muscle and appears as a hyperechoic triangular or oval-shaped structure.
- The needle should then be inserted in-plane from lateral to medial to deposit local anesthetic (20–30 mL) around the nerve under direct visualization (**Fig. 3**).

If the sciatic nerve is not easily visible at this location, it may be viewed more distally in the upper thigh between the biceps femoris and adductor magnus muscles.[16] Often, the nerve is shallower at this location. Peripheral nerve stimulation may also be used to help confirm the appropriate needle placement.

When electing to perform a sciatic block for knee surgery, providers should be mindful of the motor blockade that will likely occur, resulting in hamstring weakness and deficits in plantarflexion, dorsiflexion, eversion, and inversion of the foot.

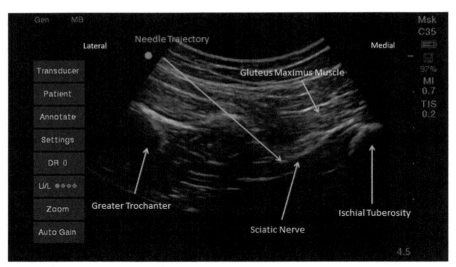

Fig. 3. Sciatic nerve block ultrasound.

Popliteal Sciatic Nerve Block

The popliteal approach to the sciatic nerve targets the nerve at its most superficial location in the popliteal fossa. This provides analgesia to the lower leg and foot with exception of the innervation provided by the saphenous nerve. Although this approach is frequently used for surgery below the knee, it has been described as an effective block for analgesia in knee surgery when used in combination with a saphenous or femoral nerve block (FNB).[17] However, because the posterior capsule of the knee is often innervated by articular branches from the sciatic nerve that branch proximally, anesthesia of the knee joint may be incomplete (**Fig. 4**).

Ultrasound-guided technique for popliteal sciatic nerve block

- At a variable distance above the popliteal crease (5–7 cm), the sciatic nerve branches into the common peroneal and tibial nerves.
- This can be visualized on ultrasound by placing a high-frequency linear probe transversely on the posterior aspect of the leg at the popliteal fossa with the patient in either the lateral decubitus, prone, or supine position with the leg bent and elevated for access behind the knee.
- The popliteal artery and vein are located at this location. The tibial nerve typically is present superficial and medial to the popliteal vein.
- The ultrasound probe is then slid proximally on the thigh until the common peroneal nerve becomes visible lateral to the tibia and begins to converge with the tibial nerve. This is the optimal position to block the nerves.
- The needle may be inserted with an in-plane approach, and local anesthetic (20–30 mL) is injected in incremental doses once the needle is placed adjacent to the nerves.

Posterior Cutaneous Nerve of the Thigh Block

If surgical anesthesia of the knee is necessary for surgery and neuraxial techniques are contraindicated or not desired, blockade of the posterior cutaneous nerve of the thigh should be considered in addition to the blocks described previously. The posterior

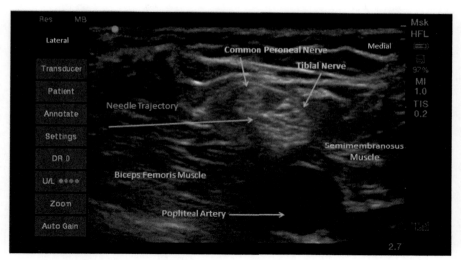

Fig. 4. Popliteal sciatic nerve block ultrasound.

cutaneous nerve of the thigh is formed from the branches of the first and second dorsal sacral rami, as well as the ventral branches of the second and third rami.[15] This nerve provides cutaneous innervation over the posterior thigh in the distribution between the lateral femoral cutaneous and anterior femoral cutaneous nerves. Blockade of this nerve can be performed by injecting 10 mL of local anesthetic to form a skin wheal just below the gluteal fold.

Femoral Nerve Block

A FNB is often performed preoperatively for orthopedic procedures involving the hip, femur, and knee to provide cutaneous and osteotome coverage. Furthermore, the FNB can be useful for providing rescue analgesia postoperatively or after acute injury.

The femoral nerve originates from the posterior division of the ventral rami of the L2-L4 nerve roots and is the largest terminal branch of the lumbar plexus. It runs lateral to the psoas muscle in the pelvis and then passes underneath the inguinal ligament to enter the anterior compartment of the thigh where it quickly branches to provide innervation to the muscles, bones, joints, and skin of the anterior thigh.[2] In the anterior thigh at the inguinal crease, the nerve is positioned 1 to 2 cm lateral to the femoral artery and vein and lies deep to the fascia lata and fascia iliaca.[18] The fascia iliaca continues underneath the femoral artery and vein providing an anatomic separation between nerve and artery (**Fig. 5**).

Ultrasound-guided technique to FNB

- FNBs are performed at the bedside with the bed flat and the patient in the supine position with legs extended.
- A high-frequency linear ultrasound transducer is placed at the femoral crease at the level of the inguinal ligament.
- The probe is slid cephalad and caudad to locate the femoral artery and vein before the division of the femoral artery into the deep and superficial branches.
- At a level before splitting of the femoral artery, the femoral nerve is identified 1 to 2 cm lateral to the artery and deep to the fascia lata and fascia iliaca.

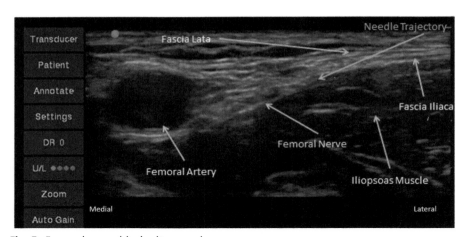

Fig. 5. Femoral nerve block ultrasound.

- An 80 to 100 mm block needle inserted in-plane, lateral to medial under ultrasound guidance, until it is under the fascia iliaca and directed toward the posterior and lateral aspect of the femoral nerve.
- After proper needle location is confirmed, local anesthetic (15–30 mL) is injected while visualizing spread underneath the fascia iliaca and surrounding the femoral nerve.

General complications and side effects shared by most peripheral nerve blocks apply to the FNB, including risk of bleeding and hematoma, infection around the injection site, neuritis, temporary or permanent nerve injury with sensory and motor involvement, and local anesthetic systemic toxicity (LAST).[19,20]

Lateral Femoral Cutaneous Nerve Block

The lateral femoral cutaneous nerve provides sensation to the anterolateral thigh, and blockade of this nerve may be used for analgesia for patients undergoing knee surgery. The lateral femoral cutaneous nerve emerges from the lateral border of the psoas major muscle and courses inferiorly and laterally toward the anterior superior iliac spine. The nerve lies deep to the fascia iliaca before it crosses the inguinal ligament toward the lateral thigh. Peripheral blockade of this nerve can be completed by landmark or ultrasound guidance.

Landmark technique for lateral femoral cutaneous block

- The landmark technique is completed by inserting a needle 2 cm medial and 2 cm inferior to the anterior superior iliac spine and injecting 5 to 10 mL of local anesthetic.

Ultrasound-guided technique for lateral femoral cutaneous block.

- The ultrasound transducer is placed inferior to the anterior superior iliac spine and at the lateral edge of the sartorius muscle.
- The lateral femoral cutaneous nerve can often be visualized between the tensor fasciae latae muscle and the sartorius muscle.
- The needle is inserted in-plane in a lateral-to-medial orientation through the subcutaneous tissue.

- Visualizing the local anesthetic in the plane between the tensor fasciae latae muscle and the sartorius muscle confirms the correct placement of the needle.

Obturator Nerve Block

The obturator nerve provides motor innervation to the adductor muscles. It also provides sensory innervation to the medial thigh and knee as described previously. The obturator nerve runs within the medial aspect of the psoas muscle and exits the pelvis by passing through the obturator foramen. The obturator nerve then divides into the anterior and posterior branches.

- The anterior branch is located between the adductor longus and adductor brevis muscles.
- The posterior branch between the fascial planes of the adductor brevis and adductor magnus muscles.

Blocking the obturator nerve can be completed under ultrasound guidance (**Fig. 6**).

Ultrasound-guided technique for obturator nerve block

- The ultrasound transducer is placed on the medial aspect of the proximal thigh.
- The anterior branch is located between the fascial planes of adductor longus and adductor brevis muscles.
- The posterior branch is located between the fascial planes of adductor brevis and adductor magnus muscles.
- The block needle is initially advanced toward the posterior branch of the obturator nerve and then toward the anterior branch. Ten to 15 mL of local anesthetic is injected at each location.

An obturator nerve block is often not necessary for adequate postoperative analgesia but must be performed for complete surgical analgesia of the knee. Risks associated with an obturator nerve block include femoral vessel puncture, nerve injury, and LAST.[15]

When motor-sparing analgesia is desired after knee surgery to allow assessment of nerve function or encourage early ambulation, the adductor canal block with or without the interspace between the popliteal artery and the capsule of the knee (IPACK) nerve blocks are suitable options. Because the innervation to the knee joint is complex and variable among patients, these nerve blocks are not reliable options for complete analgesia after surgery, but rather provide supplemental pain control in conjunction with intravenous and oral modalities.[21] The adductor canal block targets the saphenous nerve and often the posteromedial branch of the vastus medialis nerve. Block here provides analgesia to much of the knee capsule, in particular, the anteromedial and posteromedial portions. The IPACK nerve block primarily targets the articular branches of the sciatic and obturator nerves that provide sensory innervation to the posterior capsule of the knee.[22] When attempting to perform motor-sparing analgesic peripheral nerve blocks, a more dilute concentration of local anesthetic should be considered, such as 0.2% to 0.25% ropivacaine or bupivacaine.

Adductor Canal (Saphenous Nerve) Block

The saphenous nerve is purely sensory and provides innervation to the knee joint and cutaneous innervation to the medial leg and foot. In the upper leg above the knee, the saphenous nerve course alongside the femoral artery deep to the sartorius muscle. Importantly, the nerve to the vastus medialis, which provides important innervation to the medial knee joint capsule and retinaculum, is occasionally encountered in the

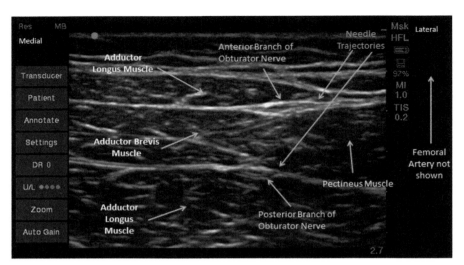

Fig. 6. Obturator nerve block.

field of view during a saphenous nerve block. This nerve occasionally lies in the subsartorial membrane lateral to the saphenous nerve and may require local anesthetic infiltration. The primary benefit of an adductor canal block over an FNB is the preservation of quadriceps muscle strength, which allows for improved function for rehabilitation and prevention of falls[23] (**Fig. 7**).

Ultrasound-guided technique for adductor canal (saphenous) nerve block

- With the patient positioned supine with leg externally rotated and slight flexion of the knee, a high-frequency linear probe is placed on the medial thigh approximately at the midpoint of the femur.
- Deep to the sartorius muscle and medial to the vastus medialis muscle lies the superficial femoral artery and corresponding saphenous nerve positioned lateral to the artery.
- The block needle is inserted in-plane and directed toward the saphenous nerve and underneath the fascial plane of the sartorius muscle.
- Local anesthetic (10–15 mL) is injected around the nerve while ensuring subsartorial spread.

IPACK Nerve Block

The primary goal of this nerve block is to infiltrate local anesthetic between the popliteal artery and the capsule of the knee. There are 2 approaches to this block with the lateral approach being discussed here. Like the adductor canal block, the primary objective of this block is to provide analgesia while maintaining motor function in the lower extremity below the knee. Infiltration of local anesthetic in this interspace will block the articular branches of the sciatic and obturator nerves that innervate the posterior capsule of the knee, which is not covered with femoral and adductor canal nerve blocks. The IPACK nerve block has consistently demonstrated a decrease in postoperative opioid equivalents immediately after surgery while avoiding sciatic nerve involvement motor blockade and the subsequent ability to ambulate after surgery[24] (**Fig. 8**).

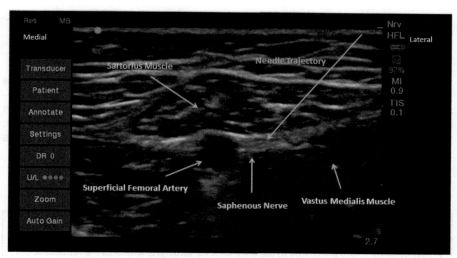

Fig. 7. Adductor canal (saphenous) nerve block.

Ultrasound-guided technique for IPACK nerve block

- With the patient positioned in the supine or lateral position with slight knee flexion, a high-frequency linear ultrasound transducer is placed slightly above the popliteal fossa to identify the distal femoral condyles, popliteal artery, and sciatic nerve.
- The block needle is inserted in-plane from the lateral aspect of the leg toward the space between the popliteal artery and the femur.
- After visualizing proper needle position, 15 to 20 mL of local anesthetic is injected in the space deep to the popliteal artery and superficial to the condyles.
- A typical injection pattern is 5 mL on the medial aspect of the popliteal artery, 5 mL directly deep the popliteal artery, and 5 mL lateral to the popliteal artery.

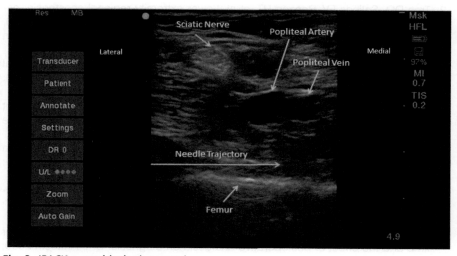

Fig. 8. IPACK nerve block ultrasound.

- The sciatic nerve branches should be visualized during the entire procedure to avoid accidental needle trauma or unintentional local anesthetic spread.

SUMMARY

The anesthetic technique for patients undergoing knee-related procedures is variable and should be tailored specifically to patient characteristics, type of injury, and surgical procedure performed. Routinely, a multimodal analgesic approach is undertaken to provide a balanced anesthetic and improve postoperative patient outcomes. Included in this multimodal approach are a variety of regional anesthetic techniques and surgical infiltration to provide adequate analgesia and motor-sparring effects.

CLINICS CARE POINTS

- Innervation of knee joint is highly variable, and consideration should be given when attempting to perform a complete surgical anesthetic of the knee.
- To provide complete anesthesia to the knee joint for surgery, branches of the femoral, sciatic, and obturator nerves, as well as the lateral femoral cutaneous nerve, must be anesthetized. This can be accomplished by targeted individual nerve blocks or neuraxial anesthesia.
- Motor-sparing analgesia of the knee can be accomplished with a combination of adductor canal saphenous and IPACK nerve blocks, as well as surgical infiltration.

DISCLOSURE

The authors have nothing to disclose.

REFERENCES

1. Tanenbaum JE, Knapik DM, Fitzgerald SJ, et al. National Incidence of Reportable Quality Metrics in the Knee Arthroplasty Population. J Arthroplasty 2017;32(10): 2941–6.
2. Tran DQ, Salinas FV, Benzon HT, et al. Lower extremity regional anesthesia: essentials of our current understanding. Reg Anesth Pain Med 2019;44(2):143–80.
3. Neal JM. Ultrasound-guided regional anesthesia and patient safety: update of an evidence-based analysis. Reg Anesth Pain Med 2016;41(2):195–204.
4. Sullivan D, Lyons M, Montgomery R, et al. Exploring opioid-sparing multimodal analgesia options in trauma: a nursing perspective. J Trauma Nurs 2016;23(6): 361–75.
5. Kukreja P, Feinstein J, Kalagara HK, et al. A summary of the anatomy and current regional anesthesia practices for postoperative pain management in total knee arthroplasty. Cureus 2018;10(6):e2755.
6. Neal JM, Barrington MJ, Brull R, et al. The second ASRA practice advisory on neurologic complications associated with regional anesthesia and pain medicine: executive summary 2015. Reg Anesth pain Med 2015;40(5):401–30.
7. Sondekoppam RV, Tsoi BC. Factors associated with risk of neurologic complications after peripheral nerve blocks: a systematic review. Anesth Analg 2017; 124(2):645–60.
8. Mar GJ, Barrington MJ, McGuirk BR. Acute compartment syndrome of the lower limb and the effect of postoperative analgesia on diagnosis. Br J Anaesth 2009; 102:3–11.

9. Kucera T, Boezaart A. Regional anesthesia does not consistently block ischemic pain: two further cases and review of the literature. Pain Med 2014;15:316–9.

10. Davis, ET, Harris A, Keene D. The use of regional anaesthesia in patients at risk of acute compartment syndrome. Inj Int J 2006;37:128–33.

11. Practice guidelines for acute pain management in the perioperative setting. Anesthesiology 2012;116(2):248–73.

12. Memtsoudis SG, Cozowicz C, Bekeris J, et al. Anaesthetic care of patients undergoing primary hip and knee arthroplasty: consensus recommendations from the International Consensus on Anaesthesia-Related Outcomes after Surgery group (ICAROS) based on a systematic review and meta-analysis. Br J Anaesth 2019; 123(3):269–87.

13. Fonkoue' L, Behets C, Kouassi JE, et al. Distribution of sensory nerves supplying the knee joint capsule and implications for genicular blockade and radiofrequency ablation: an anatomical study. Surg Radiol Anat 2019;41(12):1461–71.

14. Tran J, Peng PWH, Gofeld M, et al. Anatomical study of the innervation of posterior knee joint capsule: implication for image-guided intervention. Reg Anesth Pain Med 2019;44:234–8.

15. Hadzic A. Hadzik's textbook of regional anesthesia and acute pain management. 2nd edition. New York: McGraw-Hill Education/Medical; 2017.

16. Grant SA, Auyong DB. Ultrasound guided regional anesthesia. 2nd edition. New York: Oxford University Press; 2017.

17. Seo J, Seo S, Kim D, et al. Does combination therapy of popliteal sciatic nerve block and adductor canal block effectively control early postoperative pain after total knee arthroplasty? Knee Surg Relat Res 2017;29(4):276–81.

18. Vloka JD, Hadzić A, Drobnik L, et al. Anatomical landmarks for femoral nerve block: a comparison of four needle insertion sites. Anesth Analg 1999;89: 1467–70.

19. Sharma S, Iorio R, Specht LM, Davies-Lepie S, Healy WL. Complications of femoral nerve block for total knee arthroplasty. Clin Orthop Relat Res. 2010 Jan; 468(1): 135–140.Published online 2009 Aug 13. doi: 10.1007/s11999-009-1025-1

20. Widmer B, Lustig S, Scholes CJ, et al. Incidence and severity of complications due to femoral nerve blocks performed for knee surgery. New York: The Knee. U.S. National Library of Medicine; 2013.

21. Layera S, Aliste J, Bravo D, et al. Motor-sparing nerve blocks for total knee replacement: a scoping review. J Clin Anesth 2021;68. https://doi.org/10.1016/j.jclinane.2020.110076.

22. Tran J, Giron Arango L, Peng P, et al. Evaluation of the IPACK block injectate spread: a cadaveric study. Reg Anesth Pain Med 2019. https://doi.org/10.1136/rapm-2018-100355. rapm-2018-100355.

23. Vora M, Nicholas T, Kassel C, et al. Adductor canal block for knee surgical procedures: review article. J Clin Anesth 2016;35:295–303.

24. D'Souza RS, Langford BJ, Olsen DA, et al. Ultrasound-guided local anesthetic infiltration between the popliteal artery and the capsule of the posterior knee (IPACK) block for primary total knee arthroplasty: a systematic review of randomized controlled trials. Local Reg Anesth 2021;14:85–98.

Anesthesia for the Patient Undergoing Foot and Ankle Surgery

Christopher M. Sharrow, MD, Brett Elmore, MD*

KEYWORDS

- Foot surgery • Ankle surgery • Lower extremity nerve blocks • Sciatic block
- Saphenous block • Ankle block

KEY POINTS

- There exist several suitable anesthetic techniques for foot and ankle surgery including peripheral nerve blocks, monitored anesthesia care, general anesthesia, and neuraxial anesthesia.
- Lower extremity nerve blocks are ideally suited to provide both comprehensive postoperative analgesia and, in combination with monitored anesthesia care (MAC), anesthesia for most foot and ankle surgeries.
- Familiarity with foot and ankle innervation allows a skilled anesthesiologist to tailor the choice of peripheral nerve blocks to maximize analgesic benefit and minimize side effects.
- The ideal anesthetic involves careful evaluation of the risks and benefits of patient, surgical, and anesthetic factors.
- Multimodal analgesic agents can be used either in conjunction with regional anesthesia techniques or alone to limit postoperative pain and the side effects of opioid-only therapy.

INTRODUCTION

Foot and ankle pain affects more than 1 in 5 adults middle-aged and older and, with up to 10% of the population experiencing disabling foot pain, many seek surgical intervention to alleviate the pain.[1,2] In the Medicare population alone, it is estimated that the economic burden of foot and ankle surgery was $11 billion in 2011.[3] Increasing health care costs have led to a focus on quality and reduced lengths of stay in the hospital, shifting many foot and ankle procedures to be performed in an ambulatory surgery center (ASC). Advancements in safe anesthesia techniques, including regional anesthesia and multimodal approaches to analgesia have, in part, been responsible for a favorable safety profile for foot and ankle procedures in ASCs.[4] Here we will

Department of Anesthesiology, University of Virginia Health, PO Box 800710, Charlottesville, VA 22908-0710, USA
* Corresponding author.
E-mail address: brett.elmore@virginia.edu
Twitter: @elmorbr (B.E.)

Clin Sports Med 41 (2022) 263–280
https://doi.org/10.1016/j.csm.2021.11.010
0278-5919/22/Published by Elsevier Inc.

explore anesthesia for foot and ankle procedures, with elaboration on the anatomy underpinning the regional techniques, their ultrasound-guided technical performance, and their relative benefits and risks. We will also examine other factors that influence the anesthetic approach, such as common comorbidities associated with this population and details of the surgical procedures. After, we will include a concise review of the evidence for the use of some multimodal agents in this population. We conclude this section with the authors' recommendations on appropriate anesthesia techniques for common foot and ankle procedures.

DISCUSSION
Innervation of the Distal Lower Extremity

Sciatic nerve
The sciatic nerve (SN) is the largest branch of the lumbosacral plexus, typically arising from 4th and 5th lumbar spinal nerves as well as the 1st through 3rd sacral nerves. While the SN seems to be a single nerve in its proximal course, it is in fact, 2 individual nerves that travel together within a common connective tissue sheath: the tibial (TN) and common peroneal (or fibular) nerves (CPN). Most commonly, the SN divides into these nerves at the proximal margin of the popliteal fossa (**Fig. 1**) though significant variability is described.[5] Within the popliteal fossa, the sural nerve branches from the TN in combination with the sural communicating nerve from the CPN.

The larger TN continues posterior to the knee capsule and popliteus muscle, crossing from the lateral to the medial side of the popliteal artery. Distal to the knee (**Fig. 2**), it descends in parallel with the posterior tibial artery anterior to the gastrocnemius and soleus muscles and posterior to the tibialis posterior muscle. Just posterior to the medial malleolus, the TN branches into the calcaneal, medial, and lateral plantar nerves.

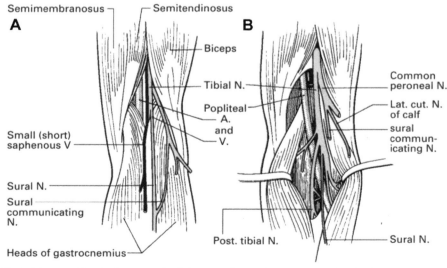

Fig.1. The popliteal fossa with (*A*) superficial dissection and (*B*) deep dissection. (Figure reprinted with permission from Lawson A, Ellis H. *Anatomy for Anaesthetists*, 9th edition, John Wiley and Sons, 2013)

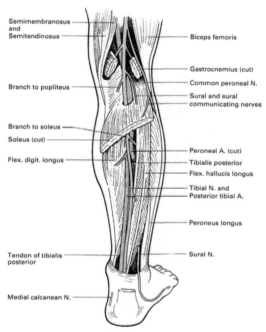

Fig. 2. The course of the tibial nerve in the calf. (Figure reprinted with permission from Lawson A, Ellis H. *Anatomy for Anaesthetists*, 9th edition, John Wiley and Sons, 2013)

Before exiting the popliteal fossa, the smaller CPN gives rise to the nerve to the short heads of the biceps, the sural communicating nerve, and the lateral cutaneous of the calf. The CPN travels laterally along the medial border of the biceps femoris, then abruptly anterior along the head of the fibula. It is along the fibular neck whereby the CPN most commonly branches into the deep and superficial peroneal nerves (DPN and SPN, respectively).

The DPN descends lateral to the tibialis anterior muscle (**Fig. 3**), traveling anterior to the extensor digitorum proximally, then anterior to the extensor hallucis longus muscle and interosseous membrane more distally before crossing the malleoli, deep to the extensor retinacula, whereby the DPN branches into its terminal medial and lateral branches innervating the dorsum of the cutaneous webspace between the 1st and 2nd toes. The anterior tibial artery can sometimes be seen crossing lateral to medial to the nerve just above the malleoli before traveling with the medial branch of the DPN to the distal foot.

The SPN travels down the distal lateral leg anterior to (and in relative parallel with) the fibula between the peroneus longus muscle and extensor digitorum longus muscles proximally, and the peroneus brevis and extensor group distally. Just proximal to the malleoli and anterior to the extensor retinacula, the SPN branches into its medial dorsal cutaneous and intermediate (sometimes called lateral) dorsal branches whereby it innervates most of the dorsum of the foot.

Saphenous nerve
The saphenous nerve (SaN) is the largest sensory branch of the femoral nerve. It arises within the femoral triangle whereby it runs lateral and parallel to the superficial femoral

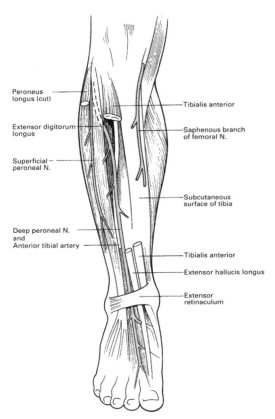

Peroneus longus (cut)

Extensor digitorum longus

Superficial peroneal N.

Deep peroneal N. and Anterior tibial artery

Tibialis anterior

Saphenous branch of femoral N.

Subcutaneous surface of tibia

Tibialis anterior

Extensor hallucis longus

Extensor retinaculum

Fig. 3. Dissection of the deep peroneal and the superficial peroneal nerve at the front of the leg. (Figure reprinted with permission from Lawson A, Ellis H. *Anatomy for Anaesthetists*, 9th edition, John Wiley and Sons, 2013)

artery. It descends into the adductor canal whereby it is bounded anteriorly by the sartorius muscle, posteriorly by the adductor longus muscle, and laterally infrapatellar branches, the distal SaN runs with the saphenous vein medial to the tibia whereby it cutaneously innervates the medial leg. It emerges anteromedially to the medial malleolus and continues to roughly the level of the navicular bone? or the first metatarsal in 80% of specimens, though it has been shown to extend into the base of first metatarsal in a minority of cadavers.[6,7]

OTHER ANATOMIC CONSIDERATIONS

Of note, it is suggested that the posterior femoral cutaneous nerve may have a role in innervating the lower leg and foot in some. In a recent cadaveric study, it was found to terminate in the distal leg in roughly 45% of cases, reaching as far as the calcaneus in one cadaver.[8] This finding may partly describe why pain can persist postoperatively despite high-quality SN and SaN blocks.

See **Table 1** for the common distal innervation of the SaN and the terminal branches of the SN. Recognize that there is anatomic variability and some conjecture by the authors in this reference.

Table 1
Distal innervation of saphenous nerve and branches of sciatic nerve

	Motor Innervation	Cutaneous Innervation	Osteotomal Innervation
Saphenous Nerve	None	Medial leg distal to knee Medial hindfoot	Medial malleolus Medial calcaneus Medial talus [a]Navicular [a]Medial cuneiform [a]1st metatarsal [a]Tarsometatarsal joint
Tibial Nerve	Tibialis posterior Flexor digitorum longus Flexor hallucis longus Soleus Interossei and lumbricals of foot	Posterior aspect of leg distal to knee Plantar surface of foot Plantar fascia	Distal fibula Distal tibia Lateral malleolus Ankle joint Plantar phalanges
Deep Peroneal Nerve	Tibialis anterior Extensor hallucis longus Extensor digitorum longus	Webspace of 1st and 2nd toe	Dorsal/lateral aspect of phalanges of 1st toe Dorsal/medial aspect of phalanges of 2nd toe
Superficial Peroneal Nerve	Peroneus longus Peroneus brevis	Anterior aspect of distal $1/3$ of leg below the knee Dorsum of foot	Dorsal surfaces of 1st-5th Phalanges [a]Talus [a]Navicular
Sural Nerve	None	Lateral leg distal to knee Lateral hind/midfoot	Lateral malleolus [a]Lateral calcaneus [a]Cuboid [a]5th metatarsal

[a] Denotes inconsistent innervation.

ULTRASOUND-GUIDED REGIONAL ANESTHETIC TECHNIQUES FOR FOOT AND ANKLE SURGERY

With an understanding of the common innervation patterns of the sciatic and SaN, an anesthesiologist can use regional anesthesia for nearly any procedure of the foot and ankle. Advantages of regional anesthetic techniques are numerous and include reduced perioperative opioid use, reduced pain scores, improved postoperative sleep, improved patient satisfaction scores, and reduced time in the postanesthesia care unit (PACU).[9–11] Here we will describe some of the most common approaches to performing ultrasound-guided peripheral nerve blocks for foot and ankle surgery.

POPLITEAL SCIATIC NERVE BLOCK

Blockade of the SN with an ultrasound-guided popliteal approach is a versatile regional anesthetic technique that is well suited for foot and ankle procedures. It provides both motor and sensory blockade of the lower limb below the knee, with the exception of the medial aspect of the lower leg and ankle, which is covered by the SaN. The popliteal sciatic block is frequently combined with a SaN block at the adductor canal to provide complete anesthesia of the distal leg, ankle, and foot. In contrast to more proximal approaches to the SN, the popliteal block spares the motor innervation to the hamstring muscles and therefore allows patients to maintain flexion at the knee.[12] This is an important advantage in ambulatory foot and ankle surgery, as it helps facilitate assisted ambulation.

The popliteal sciatic block is most commonly performed with a lateral, in-plane approach, with the patient positioned supine or lateral. If the patient is supine, the foot can be elevated on a footrest or foam block to allow for the placement of the ultrasound transducer in the popliteal crease. Alternatively, the block can be performed with a posterior approach, using either an in-plane or out-of-plane technique, with the patient in the lateral or prone position.

To perform the block, the ultrasound transducer is placed in the popliteal crease and the popliteal artery and vein are initially identified. Next, the TN is identified as a hyperechoic round or oval structure superficial and slightly lateral to the popliteal vessels.[13] The CPN is next identified as a smaller and less hyperechoic structure, typically just superficial and lateral to the TN. The transducer is then moved proximally until the 2 components of the SN are seen to join together. The block is typically performed at the level whereby the common peroneal and tibial components of the SN bifurcate, with the goal being to direct the needle between the 2 components and inject the local anesthetic within the common sciatic sheath.[13] Frequently, tilting the probe so that the beam is directed more caudally will help with the visualization of the nerves. With the needle in the correct position, the injection should result in the spread of local anesthetic within the common sciatic sheath, often separating the 2 sciatic components within.

SAPHENOUS NERVE BLOCK AT THE ADDUCTOR CANAL

Blockade of the SaN is a useful adjunct to sciatic blocks for foot and ankle procedures. The SaN provides innervation to the medial aspect of the lower leg, extending distally to the medial ankle and foot. While the SaN can be blocked at various locations along its course, a common approach, especially when paired with a popliteal sciatic block, is to perform the block at the mid-thigh level within the adductor canal.

To perform this block, the patient is positioned supine with the operative leg externally rotated. The ultrasound probe is placed transversely over the mid-thigh and the femoral artery is identified in cross-section as it passes deep to the sartorius muscle. The sartorius muscle descends in a lateral to the medial direction across the anterior thigh to form the "roof" of the adductor canal, which is bordered by vastus medialis laterally and the adductor longus and magnus medially.[14] The needle is then advanced in-plane from a lateral to medial direction, either through the sartorius muscle (trans-sartorial approach) or deep to the sartorius (sub-sartorial approach) until the needle tip lies deep to the sartorius fascia and just lateral to the superficial femoral artery. Local anesthetic should be seen spreading immediately lateral and superficial to the femoral artery, within the adductor canal. A major advantage of the SaN block is that it spares quadricep strength, relative to a femoral block. However, it is possible to cause a partial motor blockade of the vastus medialis when large volumes of anesthetic are injected subsartorially, so caution should still be taken when advising patients about unsupported ambulation following this block.[14]

ANKLE BLOCK

For surgical procedures involving the mid and distal foot, an ankle block is an effective technique to provide both surgical anesthesia and postoperative analgesia, while preserving plantar flexion and dorsiflexion at the ankle, thus allowing the patient to potentially be heel weight bearing, with assistance, immediately postoperatively.[15] While there are numerous descriptions of landmark-based approaches, the use of ultrasound has been shown to increase the clinical efficacy of ankle blocks than landmark-based techniques.[16] Given that this block requires multiple superficial injections, the authors find that intravenous moderate sedation is often an important component of performing this block comfortably for the patient. In contrast to deeper blocks, ankle blocks can be performed with smaller gauge needles (25G or 27G), which also helps to limit patient discomfort.

To perform a complete ankle block, 5 separate nerves must be anesthetized. These include the terminal branches of the SN (tibial, deep peroneal, superficial peroneal, and sural nerves) and the SaN. Each of these nerves can be blocked using either an in-plane or out-of-plane technique. Figure 4 illustrates the authors' approach to each of the individual ankle blocks with corresponding sonographic images and anatomic overlays included (**Figure 4**).

TIBIAL NERVE

The TN innervates the heel and sole of the foot and, at the level of the ankle, the TN and artery travel within the groove between the tibialis posterior and flexor digitorum longus muscles and then passes posterior to the medial malleolus. To perform the block, the ultrasound probe is placed transversely just superior and posterior to the medial malleolus. The tibial artery is first identified and can be aided with the use of color Doppler. The TN is typically seen just posterior to the artery and is intimately associated with the vessel, helping distinguish it from the surrounding tendons.[17]

DEEP PERONEAL

The DPN provides sensory innervation to the deep dorsal structures of the foot and the webspace between the first and second toes, as well as motor innervation to the ankle extensor muscles (tibialis anterior, extensor digitorum longus, and brevis, and extensor hallucis longus and brevis). To perform the block, the ultrasound probe is placed transversely at the level of the extensor retinaculum whereby the nerve is typically just medial or just lateral to the anterior tibial artery. The nerve can often be

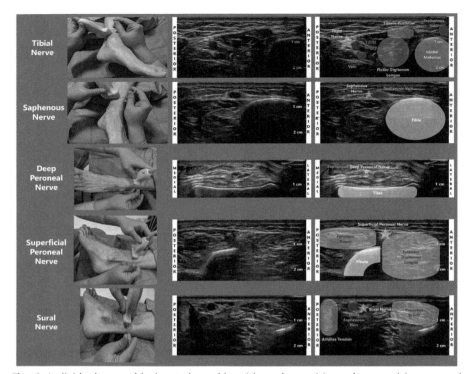

Fig. 4. Individual nerve blocks at the ankle with probe position, ultrasound image, and anatomic identifiers.

difficult to distinguish from the surrounding tissue, so a common practice is to deposit local anesthetic on either side of the anterior tibial artery.[17]

SUPERFICIAL PERONEAL NERVE

The SPN provides sensory innervation to the dorsal aspect of the foot and motor innervation to the peroneus longus and brevis muscles. It travels in the lateral compartment of the leg between the peroneus longus and extensor digitorum longus muscles.[18] To perform the block, the ultrasound probe is placed transversely over the antero-lateral aspect of the distal lower leg. To help with identification of the nerve, the prominent groove between the extensor digitorum longus and peroneal brevis muscle extending from the fibula is first identified. More proximally, the nerve runs in this groove, just deep to the fascia.[17] As it is traced distally, the nerve emerges from the fascia to lie in the subcutaneous tissue. The block can be performed at any point along this course. Performing the block more proximally can be advantageous in cases of distal edema or infection and may be less painful than subcutaneous infiltration distally.[18]

SURAL NERVE

The sural nerve provides sensory innervation to the lateral aspect of the foot and ankle and travels along the lateral border of the Achilles tendon, passing posterior to the lateral malleolus. The sural nerve is frequently in the immediate vicinity of the small saphenous vein and this vessel can serve as an important landmark. To perform the block, the transducer is placed transversely, just posterior to the lateral malleolus, and the small saphenous vein is first identified. Using light probe pressure, as well as a calf tourniquet can help facilitate visualization of the vein, which is easily compressible.[17] The sural nerve is typically seen as a small hyperechoic structure intimately associated with the small saphenous vein.

SAPHENOUS NERVE

The SaN innervates the medial malleolus and a variable portion of the medial hind and midfoot. It is a small nerve that travels down the medial aspect of the leg, in close proximity to the greater saphenous vein, and is often difficult to visualize. As such, the saphenous vein is typically used as a landmark. To perform the block, the transducer is placed over the distal, anterior-medial aspect of the leg and the saphenous vein is identified. Again, gentle probe pressure, along with a calf tourniquet, can be used to help facilitate visualization of the vein.[17] Injection of local anesthetic around this vessel, in the authors' experience, results in reliable blockade of the nerve.

CONTINUOUS CATHETER TECHNIQUES

While single-injection peripheral nerve blocks offer many advantages, the benefits are inherently limited by the duration of the local anesthetic used. Using a continuous peripheral nerve block technique offers the ability to prolong the beneficial effects of the nerve block beyond the initial postoperative hours and has been shown to decrease postoperative pain, decrease the use of opioid pain medication and improve patient satisfaction following painful orthopedic foot and ankle procedures.[10] In addition, the use of portable mechanical and elastomeric pumps for the infusion of local anesthetic can allow patients to continue to receive these benefits after leaving the hospital. In a prospective trial of 30 patients undergoing moderately painful orthopedic surgery of the lower extremity, Ilfeld and colleagues demonstrated that patients who went home with a popliteal SN catheter infusion of 0.2% ropivacaine showed decreased pain, decreased opioid use and opioid-related side effects, decreased sleep disturbances and improved overall satisfaction.[11]

When placing a popliteal sciatic catheter, there are potential advantages of using a lateral approach, as opposed to a posterior approach. With a lateral approach, the catheter passes through the biceps femoris muscle, which may help to stabilize the catheter and prevent dislodgement, compared with the subcutaneous tissue of the posterior popliteal fossa. In addition, securing the catheter on the lateral thigh results in less movement of the surrounding tissue with knee flexion and extension, again helping to limit the chances of dislodgement.[13] Lastly, securing the catheter laterally provides more convenient access to the insertion site for both the clinician and patient.

In addition, continuous SaN catheters can be used in conjunction with sciatic catheters and may be particularly useful for procedures involving the medial aspect of the ankle. This dual catheter technique, consisting of both a popliteal sciatic and saphenous catheter, has been shown to reduce pain scores, improve satisfaction with pain control and reduce opioid use in the early postoperative period.[19]

COMPLICATIONS FROM LOWER EXTREMITY NERVE BLOCKS

Low complication rates with regional anesthesia have been consistently demonstrated in large prospective and retrospective, as well as meta-analyses.[20] Potential complications of any regional techniques include local anesthetic toxicity, infection, bleeding, hematoma formation, and nerve injury. A prospective, observational study by Kahn and colleagues in 2017 looked at the incidence of neurologic and peripheral nerve block site complications in 2704 patients at a busy center that used both popliteal sciatic and ankle blocks.[21] While they found an overall complication rate of 7.2%, the rate of serious neurologic complications was much lower at 0.7%, with an unclear etiology in most cases. In addition, while they found a higher overall complication rate for popliteal blocks (8.8%) than ankle blocks (2.5%), the study authors felt that the true complication rates were ultimately similar once obvious patient confounders were accounted for.[21] Thus, these data looking specifically at rates of complications with peripheral nerve blocks for foot and ankle surgery were similar to previously reported rates of serious neurologic complications with peripheral nerve blocks and provide evidence for the relative safety and efficacy of these techniques.

MULTIMODAL ANALGESIA

Poorly controlled pain following foot and ankle surgery significantly impacts patient outcomes and has been associated with unplanned hospital admissions from outpatient facilities, prolonged time in the postoperative care unit, delayed discharge to home, and delayed return to normal activities.[22] A plan for successful postoperative analgesia is a crucial component of the overall anesthetic plan and can be made in conjunction with the patient and the surgeon, taking into consideration patient-specific comorbidities, anticipated postoperative pain, plans for ambulation and surgeon and facility preferences and capabilities.

A multimodal approach to postoperative analgesia offers the advantage of improving pain control and limiting the side effects of individual interventions by combining lower doses of agents with different mechanisms of action. When possible, regional anesthetic techniques (either single injection or continuous infusion) are generally favored as the cornerstone of analgesic plans for foot and ankle surgery and can be supplemented with oral or intravenous analgesics. However, in instances whereby regional techniques are not feasible or not desired by the patient, a multimodal approach to analgesia becomes especially important.

Wang and colleagues performed a systematic review of randomized controlled trials regarding analgesia for foot and ankle surgery and proposed an evidence-based template for elective procedures that included preoperative peripheral nerve block combined with oral acetaminophen plus NSAIDS or COX-2 selective inhibitors, intraoperative intravenous dexamethasone and postoperative acetaminophen and NSAIDS/COX-2 inhibitors combined with oral opioids for moderate to severe postoperative pain.[22] With the most clinically significant and well-known side effects stemming from perioperative opioids, such a multimodal approach focuses on limiting opioid use with the goal of reducing detrimental side effects, while still providing effective pain control. Such a template can be easily modified based on patient considerations, as well as individual practitioner or institutional preferences.

OVERVIEW OF FACTORS AFFECTING APPROACH TO ANESTHESIA

Any procedure of the foot and ankle can be approached with a variety of anesthetic techniques. Like other orthopedic procedures of the extremities, the predictable innervation patterns of the foot and ankle have led to the utilization of peripheral nerve blocks as a safe, efficacious, and reliable technique for both anesthesia and analgesia. Still, general anesthesia will always have utility in this arena in providing complete intraoperative comfort for the patient and optimizing the surgical field for the surgeon. The choice of anesthetic should be determined after careful consideration of factors including (but not limited to) patient comorbidities, surgical approach, surgeon preference, need for tourniquet, duration of procedure, degree of postoperative pain, postoperative ambulation needs, and presence of anticoagulation or coagulopathy. Here we will review some of these variables.

PATIENT COMORBIDITIES
Obesity and Obstructive Sleep Apnea

Obesity, whereby body mass index calculates greater than 30 kg/m^2, complicates all aspects of patient care. As the prevalence of obesity increases worldwide, so, too, does the number of patients presenting for foot and ankle surgery with concomitant obesity. Obese patients should be carefully screened for comorbid conditions such as obstructive sleep apnea (OSA), presence of difficult airway, and presence of other significant cardiopulmonary diseases that may dictate the choice of anesthetic and appropriateness for discharge to home. While all anesthetics have been used safely in all obesity classifications, regional and neuraxial techniques should be prioritized due to their ability to provide long-lasting, opioid-sparing, minimally respiratory-depressing analgesia throughout the postoperative period.[23] Although peripheral nerve blocks are expected to be more difficult in patients with an obese habitus, the risk-benefit analysis tends to tip favorably for regional anesthesia. The choice of general anesthesia versus sedation after regional anesthesia techniques is not always clear. Anticipated need for deep sedation in the presence of severe OSA suggests general anesthesia may be safer. Conversely, a relaxed patient with a dense peripheral nerve block may do well with only mild sedation. Using a patient's home continuous positive airway pressure (CPAP) device intraoperatively may be beneficial, but modern anesthesia machines can emulate CPAP machines with the added benefit of supplemental oxygenation, while also facilitating quick conversion to general anesthesia.

Preexisting Neuropathy

The presence of preexisting neuropathy may deter some anesthesiologists from pursuing regional anesthesia secondary to the fear of theoretically increased neurotoxicity based on a so-called "double crush" hypothesis. Unfortunately, the most common cause of acquired systemic polyneuropathy is diabetes mellitus, which is a frequently encountered comorbidity in the foot and ankle population. Animal models suggest that diabetic nerves are potentially more sensitive to neural injury.[24] However, the incidence of chronic nerve injury after regional anesthesia in this population is unclear, with only one study from 2006 finding 0.4% of patients with preexisting neuropathy developing new neurologic deficits after regional or neuraxial anesthesia.[25] Evidence is limited mostly to case reports in determining the safety of pursuing nerve blocks in patients with preexisting neurologic conditions.[26] A thorough preoperative neurologic examination should be performed and documented on any patient with diabetes mellitus or a diagnosis of any class of neuropathy. Decisions to perform regional anesthesia should be made on an individual basis after a thorough discussion of risks and benefits.

Restless Leg Syndrome

Few patient factors can confound successful MAC in foot and ankle surgery more than restless leg syndrome (RLS). RLS is characterized by unpleasant or tingling sensations in the legs (less commonly, the arms) especially at rest, resulting in the urge to move the extremities to relieve the sensation. When the movements occur during sleep, with or without arousal from sleep, they are known as periodic limb movements of sleep (PLMS). Interestingly, sedating medications do not seem to relieve the sensation or

PLMS and, in fact, can unmask or worsen the condition. General anesthesia seems to obliterate the leg movements, thus improving the surgical field, but worsening of RLS-associated discomfort postoperatively has been described.[27] Frequently, patients are prescribed dopamine agonists for symptomatic relief. Dopamine and histamine antagonists, such as metoclopramide, droperidol, promethazine, and diphenhydramine, should be avoided if possible. If a patient carries a diagnosis of (or symptoms consistent with) RLS, discuss the risk of this interfering with the surgical procedure. The authors note a high rate of conversion to general anesthesia when attempting to use MAC or block as primary anesthetic in patients with RLS.

Surgical Considerations

The planned site of the surgical incision and patient position needed to facilitate that incision are both important factors in determining anesthetic needs. For instance, while an SN block alone frequently provides excellent analgesia and anesthesia during an Achilles tendon repair, the procedure is most frequently performed in the prone position. Many anesthesiologists do not have comfort with MAC or block as primary anesthetic techniques in the prone position, necessitating general anesthesia. Other procedures of the foot and ankle, such as bi- and trimalleolar fracture ORIF vary in surgical preference for the patient position (supine vs prone). Communication and an understanding of your surgical colleagues' preferences are key in providing safe anesthesia for these patients.

Furthermore, given the rich innervation of the foot, some elective foot and ankle procedures are associated with higher rates of iatrogenic nerve injury.[28] While most of these injuries tend to be transient, understandably, some surgeons may prefer deferring regional anesthesia until postoperatively to assess for surgical nerve injury. A comprehensive list of common procedures and their associated iatrogenic nerve injuries are too numerous to list here, but special attention should be given to certain procedures. Anterior ankle arthroscopy has been associated with cutaneous nerve injury (up to 8.6% in older studies), most commonly from a branch of the SPN.[29–31] Additionally, total ankle arthroplasty is associated with an overall rate of nerve injury of 1.3%, most commonly in SPN or DPN distribution (0%–17.1% and 0%–12.9%, respectively).[28,32]

Tourniquet Use

Arterial tourniquets are used to limit surgical bleeding in many foot and ankle procedures. While automated pneumatic tourniquets are most frequently used, others elect to use a manually wound Esmarch bandage, particularly in forefoot surgery. While the use of Esmarch bandage has been demonstrated to be safe when used correctly,[33] it should be noted that the Esmarch bandage can generate pressures greater than 1000 mm Hg.[34] Though safe in short intervals, the use of pneumatic arterial tourniquets above the knee longer than 120 minutes is associated with CPN injury.[35] While the full pathophysiology of tourniquet pain is not completely understood, it is likely mediated by unmyelinated C-fibers that are not as responsive to local anesthetic blockade of signals (when compared with myelinated A-fibers).[36,37] Fortunately, much like peripheral nerve blocks, the risk of permanent nerve injury from tourniquet use is thought to be rare (1:3752 for lower limb procedures).[38] Many well-intentioned anesthesiologists tailor their nerve blocks to provide 'coverage' at the site of the tourniquet application, but, despite comprehensive nerve blocks, patients can still experience tourniquet pain. It is not the authors' intention to dissuade other anesthesiologists from using peripheral nerve blocks to improve patient tolerance of the tourniquet, but it should be noted that, while the hemodynamic effects

Table 2
Recommendations for blocks and anesthesia type for common procedures of the foot and ankle

	Regional Techniques	General Anesthesia vs Monitored Anesthesia Care	Other Considerations
Ankle or Leg Procedures	Surgical approaches too high to be covered by conventional ankle block	Typically a question of whether the patient is supine or prone	Polytrauma may dictate anesthetic in the case of fractures
Bi- or trimalleolar fractures	*Sciatic and Saphenous*	GA (if prone) or MAC (if supine and patient tolerates)	
Ankle arthrodesis or arthroplasty	*Sciatic and Saphenous*	GA or MAC	Duration of procedure can limit tolerance of MAC
Triple arthrodesis	*Sciatic and Saphenous*	GA or MAC	Duration of procedure can limit tolerance of MAC
Achilles tendon	*Sciatic (+/− Saphenous)*	GA (typically a prone procedure)	
Gastrocnemius recession	*Sciatic (+/− Saphenous)*	GA (typically a prone procedure)	
Mid- or Hindfoot Procedures	Saphenous nerve innerv.medial bones/joints of hind-/midfoot	Depends on density of block and patient tolerance	
Lisfranc dislocation	*Sciatic and Saphenous vs* Ankle: SPN, DPN, Saphenous, TN	GA or MAC in motivated patient	
Calcaneus fracture		GA or MAC in motivated patient	Often after fall from extreme height, may have polytrauma
5th metatarsal fracture	*Ankle: SPN, Sural, TN vs Sciatic*	MAC vs GA	"Jones fracture"
Tarsal tunnel release	*Local infiltration*	MAC vs GA	Preexisting tibial nerve dysfunction, soft tissue procedure

(continued on next page)

Table 2
(continued)

	Regional Techniques	General Anesthesia vs Monitored Anesthesia Care	Other Considerations
Broström procedure	*Sciatic* (+/– Saphenous)	GA or MAC in motivated patient	Recurrent ankle sprains, thigh tourniquet frequently
Forefoot Procedures	Ankle block ideal for most forefoot procedures	MAC well tolerated for most	Esmarch tourniquet frequently used
Hallux valgus (Akin/Chevron)	*Ankle: SPN, DPN, TN*	MAC vs GA	
1st metatarsophalangeal arthrodesis	*Ankle: SPN, DPN, TN*	MAC vs GA	
Toe/transmetatarsal amputation	*Ankle: SPN, DPN, TN,* +/– Sural (for TMA) or digital block	MAC vs GA	Ankle block nerves depends on amputated digit
Morton neuroma	*Local infiltration* vs Ankle: SPN, TN	MAC vs GA	
Weil osteotomy(ies)	*Ankle: SPN, DPN, TN*	MAC vs GA	Often combined with other procedures

of tourniquet pain can be blunted, the only modality that reliably improves a patient's tolerance of tourniquet pain is tourniquet deflation.[34] Still, a combination of peripheral nerve block techniques and/or sedation is frequently successful in facilitating patient tolerance of the arterial tourniquet at our institution, though it should be expected that a significant number of patients will require conversion to general anesthesia partly because of tourniquet intolerance.

Anticoagulation/Coagulopathy

In the 21st century, a wide array of anticoagulants exists to reduce thromboembolic events. In addition to the vitamin K antagonist, warfarin, and platelet aggregation inhibitors, such as aspirin and clopidogrel, patients are more frequently taking novel direct oral anticoagulants. These include direct factor Xa inhibitors such as apixaban and rivaroxaban, and direct thrombin inhibitors, such as argatroban. Careful attention should be paid to a patient's anticoagulation regimen before using neuraxial or regional anesthesia. Understandably, it may be difficult for anesthesiologists to remember the half-lives of these agents and the safe windows of invasive procedures after cessation of the drugs. As a comprehensive summary of recommendations would be too lengthy to include here, the authors recommend using the American Society of Regional Anesthesia (ASRA) Coags App, available for $3.99 on your smartphone in both the Apple App and Google Play stores. The app allows for the quick assessment of the ASRA recommendations for using regional anesthesia in the patient on anticoagulation therapy, published in 2018.[39] This becomes especially useful for determining the safety of neuraxial procedures. Broadly, however, the approaches for the peripheral nerve blocks we list here all fall within anatomically compressible areas of the body. The ASRA anticoagulation guidelines suggest managing these blocks based on their compressibility, vascularity, and the consequences of bleeding (grade 2C evidence).[39]

The authors apply this recommendation when evaluating the risks and benefits of peripheral techniques in the anticoagulated or coagulopathic patient.

SUMMARY

The anesthetic approach to any unique surgical procedure of the foot and ankle will vary greatly depending on anesthesiologist, surgeon, and patient factors. With that understanding, the authors make recommendations on regional anesthesia techniques based on the surgical procedure in **Table 2**.

CLINICS CARE POINTS

- As the CPN passes below the knee and around the fibular head, it lies very superficially, protected only by skin and superficial fascia. It is at this location that the nerve is particularly vulnerable to pressure injury resulting from surgical positioning. Such pressure injuries can lead to postoperative CPN neuropraxia.

- The popliteal approach to the SN, in contrast to more proximal approaches, spares the motor innervation to the hamstring muscles and therefore allows patients to maintain flexion at the knee. This is an important advantage in ambulatory foot and ankle surgery, as it helps facilitate assisted ambulation.

- When performing a sciatic nerve block, minor adjustments in the angle of the probe can often enhance the visibility of the nerve and its components, with a more caudad beam angle frequently yielding more distinct images of the neural structures.

- When performing SaN and sural nerve blocks at the ankle, the greater saphenous and small saphenous veins, respectively, are important landmarks. Identification of these easily compressible vessels can be assisted by the use of gentle probe pressure, as well as the use of an ankle tourniquet.
- The use of a multimodal approach to pharmacologic postoperative analgesia is especially important in instances whereby a regional technique cannot be performed.
- Lower extremity arterial tourniquet times in excess of 120 minutes have been associated with CPN injury, so efforts should be made to track and limit these times, when possible.

DISCLOSURE

The authors have nothing to disclose.

REFERENCES

1. Thomas MJ, Roddy E, Zhang W, et al. The population prevalence of foot and ankle pain in middle and old age: A systematic review. Pain 2011;152(12):2870–80.
2. Garrow AP, Silman AJ, Macfarlane GJ. The cheshire foot pain and disability survey: A population survey assessing prevalence and associations. Pain 2004;110(1–2):378–84.
3. Belatti DA, Phisitkul P. Economic burden of foot and ankle surgery in the US medicare population. Foot Ankle Int 2014;35(4):334–40.
4. Adamson P, Peters W, Janney C, et al. The safety of foot and ankle procedures at an ambulatory surgery center. J Orthopaedics 2020;21:203–6.
5. Vloka JD, Hadžic A, April E, et al. The Division of the Sciatic Nerve in the Popliteal Fossa: Anatomical Implications for Popliteal Nerve Blockade. Anesth Analg 2001;92(1):215–7.
6. Aszmann OC, Ebmer JM, Dellon AL. Cutaneous Innervation of the Medial Ankle: An Anatomic Study of the Saphenous, Sural, and Tibial Nerves and their Clinical Significance. Foot Ankle Int 1998;19(11):753–6.
7. Marsland D, Dray A, Little NJ, et al. The saphenous nerve in foot and ankle surgery: Its variable anatomy and relevance. Foot Ankle Surg 2013;19(2):76–9.
8. Feigl GC, Schmid M, Zahn PK, et al. The posterior femoral cutaneous nerve contributes significantly to sensory innervation of the lower leg: an anatomical investigation. Br J Anaesth 2020;124(3):308–13.
9. Collins L, Bao Ffarcsi B, Halwani A, et al. Impact of a regional anesthesia analgesia program for outpatient foot surgery. Can J Anesthesiol 1999;46(9):840–5.
10. White PF, Issioui T, Skrivanek GD, et al. The use of a continuous popliteal sciatic nerve block after surgery involving the foot and ankle: does it improve the quality of recovery? Anesth Analg 2003;97(5):1303–9.
11. Ilfeld BM, Morey TE, Doris Wang R, et al. Continuous Popliteal Sciatic Nerve Block for Postoperative Pain Control at Home. Anesthesiology 2002;97(4):959–65.
12. Hebl J, Jacob A. Chapter 27: Popliteal blockade. In: Hebl J, Lennon R, editors. Mayo Clinic Atlas of Regional Anesthesia and Ultrasound-Guided Nerve Blockade. New York, NY: Oxford University Press; 2010. p. 423–41.
13. Hadzic A, et al. Chapter 33G: Ultrasound-guided popliteal sciatic block. In: Hadzic A, editor. Hadzic's Textbook of Regional Anesthesia and Acute Pain Management. 2nd edition. New York, NY: McGraw-Hill Education; 2017. p. 628–35.

14. Bendtsen TF, Lopez AM, Clark TB. Chapter 33E: Ultrasound-guided saphenous (subsartorius/adductor canal) nerve block. In: Hadzic A, editor. Hadzic's Textbook of Regional Anesthesia. 2nd. New York, NY: McGraw Hill Education; 2017. p. 615–9.
15. Gray AT. Chapter 46: Ankle block, . Atlas of Ultrasound-Guided Regional Anesthesia. 2nd edition. Philadelphia, PA: El Sevier Saunders; 2012. p. 194.
16. Chin KJ, Wong NWY, MacFarlane AJR, et al. Ultrasound-guided versus anatomic landmark-guided ankle blocks: A 6-year retrospective review. Reg Anesth Pain Med 2011;36(6):611–8.
17. Vandepitte C, et al. Chapter 33H: Ultrasound-guided ankle block. In: Hadzic A, editor. Hadzic's Textbook of Regional Anesthesia. 2nd. New York, NY: McGraw-Hill Education; 2017. p. 636–41.
18. Gray AT. Chapter 48: Superficial peroneal nerve block. In: Gray AT, editor. Atlas of Ultrasound-Guided Regional Anesthesia. 2nd. Philadelphia, PA: Elsevier Saunders; 2016. p. 201–7.
19. Jarrell K, McDonald E, Shakked R, et al. Combined popliteal catheter with single-injection vs continuous-infusion saphenous nerve block for foot and ankle surgery. Foot Ankle Int 2018;39(3):332–7.
20. Pearce CJ, Hamilton PD. Current concepts review: Regional anesthesia for foot and ankle surgery. Foot Ankle Int 2010;31(8):732–9.
21. Kahn RL, Ellis SJ, Cheng J, et al. The incidence of complications is low following foot and ankle surgery for which peripheral nerve blocks are used for postoperative pain management. HSS J 2018;14(2):134–42.
22. Wang J, Liu GT, Mayo HG, et al. Pain Management for Elective Foot and Ankle Surgery: A Systematic Review of Randomized Controlled Trials. J Foot Ankle Surg 2015;54(4):625–35.
23. Memtsoudis SG, Cozowicz C, Nagappa M, et al. Society of anesthesia and sleep medicine guideline on intraoperative management of adult patients with obstructive sleep apnea. Anesth Analg 2018;127(4):967–87.
24. Kalichman MW, Calcutt NA. Local anesthetic-induced conduction block and nerve fiber injury in streptozotocin-diabetic rats. Anesthesiology 1992;77(5): 941–7.
25. Hebl JR, Kopp SL, Schroeder DR, et al. Neurologic complications after neuraxial anesthesia or analgesia in patients with preexisting peripheral sensorimotor neuropathy or diabetic polyneuropathy. Anesth Analg 2006;103(5):1294–9.
26. Kopp SL, Jacob AK, Hebl JR. Regional Anesthesia in Patients with Preexisting Disease. Reg Anesth Pain Med 2015;40:467–78. https://doi.org/10.1097/AAP.0000000000000179.
27. Ohshita N, Yamagata K, Himejima A, et al. Anesthetic management of a patient with restless legs syndrome: a case report. Anesth Prog 2020;67(4):226–9.
28. Veljkovic A, Dwyer T, Lau JT, et al. Neurological complications related to elective orthopedic surgery: part 3: common foot and ankle procedures. Reg Anesth Pain Med 2015;40(5):455–66.
29. Deng DF, Hamilton GA, Lee M, et al. Complications Associated with Foot and Ankle Arthroscopy. J Foot Ankle Surg 2012;51(3):281–4.
30. Zengerink M, van Dijk CN. Complications in ankle arthroscopy. Knee Surg Sports Traumatol Arthrosc 2012;20(8):1420–31.
31. Martin DF, Baker CL, Curl WW, et al. Operative ankle arthroscopy: Long-term followup. Am J Sports Med 1989;17(1):16–23.
32. Zaidi R, Cro S, Gurusamy K, et al. The outcome of total ankle replacement: A systematic review and meta-analysis. Bone Joint J 2013;95 B(11):1500–7.

33. Grebing BR, Coughlin MJ. Evaluation of the Esmark Bandage as a Tourniquet for Forefoot Surgery. Foot Ankle Int 2004;25(6):397–405.
34. van der Spuy L. Complications of the arterial tourniquet. South Afr J Anaesth Analgesia 2012;18(1):14–8.
35. Horlocker TT, Hebl JR, Gali B, et al. Anesthetic, patient, and surgical risk factors for neurologic complications after prolonged total tourniquet time during total knee arthroplasty. Anesth Analg 2006;102(3):950–5.
36. Concepcion MA, Lambert DH, Welch KA, et al. Tourniquet pain during spinal anesthesia: a comparison of plain solutions of tetracaine and bupivacaine. Anesth Analg 1988;67:828–32.
37. Gissen A, Covino B, Gregus J. Differential sensitivities of mammalian nerve fibers to local anesthetic agents. Anesthesiology 1980;53:467–74.
38. Mingo-Robinet J, Castañeda-Cabrero C, Alvarez V, et al. Tourniquet-related iatrogenic femoral nerve palsy after knee surgery: case report and review of the literature. Case Rep Orthopedics 2013;2013:1–4.
39. Horlocker TT, Wedel DJ, Rowlingson JC, et al. Regional Anesthesia in the patient receiving antithrombotic or thrombolytic therapy; American Society of Regional Anesthesia and Pain Medicine evidence-based guidelines (Third Edition). Reg Anesth Pain Med 2010;35(1):64–101.

Safety Considerations for Outpatient Arthroplasty

Alberto E. Ardon, MD, MPH

KEYWORDS

- Safety • Outpatient • Arthroplasty • Same-day discharge

KEY POINTS

- Patients undergoing outpatient arthroplasty may be at increased risk of complications.
- Appropriate patient selection is critical for success and safety in outpatient arthroplasty.
- Potential exclusion criteria for outpatient arthroplasty may include age greater than 75 years, bleeding disorder, deep vein thrombosis, uncontrolled diabetes mellitus, and hypoalbuminemia.
- Risks of same-day versus next-day discharge may not be equivalent.

INTRODUCTION

Total joint arthroplasties (TJAs) are some of the most commonly performed major orthopedic procedures. Over the course of the previous decade, the number of total knee arthoplasties (TKA) and total hip arthroplasties (THA) performed per year has continued to increase. For example, it is estimated that by 2040, more than 300,000 TKAs will be performed annually in the United States.[1] As the removal of TKAs and THAs from the Centers for Medicare and Medicaid Services (CMS) inpatient-only list in 2018 and 2020, respectively, the number of arthroplasties performed on an outpatient basis has dramatically increased. Same-day or next-day discharge after arthroplasty has been postulated to provide cost and patient satisfaction benefits when compared with the traditional inpatient approach. For example, one study by Rosinsky and colleagues suggested a potential lifetime cost savings of USD 4867 to 8455 with an outpatient approach to total hip arthroplasties, as well as an advantage in quality-adjusted life years.[2] Concurrently, some data have suggested that outpatient arthroplasties do not pose an increased risk of complications compared with inpatient procedures. However, both surgeon and anesthesiologist should be aware

Financial Disclosures: None.
Conflicts of Interest: None.
Department of Anesthesiology and Perioperative Medicine, Mayo Clinic, 4500 San Pablo Road, Jacksonville, FL 32224, USA
E-mail address: ardon.alberto@mayo.edu

of the implications for the safety of outpatient TJAs and potential patient risk factors that could alter this safety profile.

DISCUSSION
Potential Safety of Outpatient Total Joint Arthroplasties

Several studies have been conducted on the relative safety of outpatient TJA. Unfortunately, data suggesting that outpatient arthroplasty does not have an increased risk of complications come from smaller, retrospective assessments. For example, one study by Keulen and colleagues examining 525 THA, TKA, and uni-compartment knee arthroplasty patients found no difference in the 90-day complication rate and readmission rate between 415 patients discharged on the procedure day compared with the 110 patients requiring one or more night's stay.[3] Importantly, however, specific selection criteria existed for outpatients, and outpatients were more likely to have a lower American Society of Anesthesiologists (ASA) classification (ASA class 2 or below 98% vs 94%, respectively, $P<.001$). In another retrospective case series of 400 patients with TKA, no differences in either emergency department visits or readmissions within 90 days were observed between same-day discharge patients and inpatients. However, the outpatients were younger, leaner, and had less morbidity burden.[4] Similarly, data collected from 183 patients undergoing outpatient revision knee or hip arthroplasty at a single surgical center showed a statistically similar rate of emergency department visits within 90 days of surgery compared with a similar and equally-sized inpatient cohort (3.4% vs 6.7%, respectively, $P = .214$).[5] In contrast to previously mentioned studies, the outpatients in this investigation had similar mean age, ASA class, and body mass index (BMI) compared with inpatients; they also showed no difference in postoperative admission rates. Finally, one matched case–control study querying the American Hip Institute registry found no differences regarding 2-year revision rates when comparing younger, healthier outpatients to inpatient matched controls.[6]

Risk of Adverse Events

In spite of these results, larger studies suggest that complication rates after outpatient arthroplasty may match or exceed those of inpatients. One meta-analysis examining 8 articles (comprising 212,632 patients) found that, while there was no difference in readmission rate, the overall risk ratio for any complication favored an inpatient approach.[7] Arshi and colleagues compared 4391 outpatient TKAs (defined as same-day or next-day discharge) to 128,951 inpatient TKAs in the national Humana database. After matching patients based on Charlson comorbidity index, outpatients had a higher risk of explantation (odds ratio (OR):1.3) tibial/femoral component revision (OR: 1.22), incision and drainage (OR: 1.5), deep venous thromboembolism (DVT) (OR: 1.42), and need for postoperative knee manipulation (OR: 1.28).[8] A recent Surgeons National Surgical Quality Improvement Program (NSQIP) database investigation matched 1099 outpatient TKA patients (length of stay <24 hours) to 1099 inpatients and found risk of certain adverse events (such as thromboembolism or return to the operating room) to be statistically the same between the 2 groups.[9] However, the relative risk of *any* serious adverse event was 1.82 [(0.58–3.06), $P = .005$] when comparing outpatients to inpatients. Notably, patients in the outpatient cohort (and thus in the inpatient cohort by matching) tended to be younger and with less comorbidity burden than patients who may frequently present for arthroplasty. This potential higher risk of any serious adverse event even with careful patient selection reaffirms the belief that physicians should not only be aware of potential risks but also implement protocols and pathways to miti-gate these risks even among younger and healthier patients in the ambulatory setting. For example, adherence to a strict thromboprophylaxis protocol could be emphasized by providing rigorous preoperative patient education and ensuring an adequate supply of low molecular weight heparin or anticoagulation of choice.

Risk Factors

Large-scale investigations have suggested potential risk factors for postoperative complications after outpatient arthroplasty. In one study by Sher and colleagues, age greater than 80, bleeding disorder, history of smoking, and ASA 3 or 4 classifica-tion were associated with a higher risk of unplanned admission or postdischarge se-vere adverse event after same-day or next-day discharge after arthroplasty.[10] In another study which examined 169,406 patients in the NSQIP database who under-went TKA or THA, male gender, BMI greater than 35, smoking history, and albumin less than 3.5 g/dL were found to be risk factors for return to the operating room within 30 days after surgery.[11] Interestingly, outpatient surgery was not a risk factor compared with inpatient surgery, possibly suggesting that poor preoperative patient status, regardless of setting, is a key consideration when assessing the risk of post-operative complications. Similarly (albeit after total shoulder arthroplasty), a recent study by Burton and colleagues suggested that, in addition to advanced age, bleeding disorder, and higher ASA class, the presence of congestive heart failure (OR: 3.18) or poor overall functional status (OR: 2.8) also increased the risk of unplanned admission.

Patient Selection

Given the above considerations, appropriate patient selection should be at the fore-front of the physician's mind when considering patients for outpatient arthroplasty. While national society guidelines have yet to be developed, some studies have sug-gested potential inclusion/exclusion criteria for outpatient TKA and THA. One study by Sayeed and colleagues suggested patients be less than 75 years of age and be ASA class 1 or 2.[12] Other potential exclusion criteria based on this study are listed in **Box 1**. While the presence of only one of these criteria may not be an absolute contraindication to outpatient arthroplasty, consideration should be given to the pa-tient's overall clinical picture and the degree to which that particular comorbidity is likely to increase the risk of postoperative complications. For example, among the 7474 TJA outpatients investigated by Sher and colleagues, patients who were 80 years of age or older had an odds ratio of 4.17 (95% confidence interval (CI): 1.81–8.58) of having a severe postoperative adverse event (compared with a younger patient); pa-tients with a history of smoking had a smaller odds ratio of 1.62 (95% CI: 1.06–2.46) of the same outcome (compared with no previous smoking).[10] Thus, the particular risk incurred in a patient with either a single or a certain combination of risk factors may be too high for inclusion in the outpatient setting. Likewise, one retrospective review of 325 patients who underwent outpatient TKA showed that patients who had a lower BMI, lower STOP-BANG sleep apnea score, or absence of allergies had a greater like-lihood of same-day discharge.[13] Indeed, the importance of appropriate patient selec-tion can hardly be overstated, both in regard to patient safety and potential for appropriate and timely discharge. In one 145-patient case series of direct anterior approach THAs, patients over the age of 70, with a BMI greater than 35, or with a his-tory of DVT or PE were automatically excluded from consideration for outpatient arthroplasty. The resultant healthier patient cohort had a successful same-day discharge rate of 96%.[14] Further, a review of 34,416 patients in the NSQIP database who underwent THA suggested that healthier and younger patients selected for

Box 1
Potential exclusion criteria for outpatient arthroplasty
Age greater than 75
Bleeding disorders
Congestive heart failure
Arrhythmia
History of deep venous thrombosis or pulmonary embolus
History of significant pulmonary disease (chronic obstructive pulmonary disease, emphysema, home oxygen use)
Uncontrolled diabetes mellitus (Hemoglobin A1C >7)
BMI greater than 35
History of chronic pain requiring opioids, substance abuse, or severe uncontrolled postoperative pain
Chronic renal disease (Stage 4, glomerular filtration rate <30)
Poor comprehension or unreasonable patient expectations
Albumin less than 3.5 g/dL
Adapted from Sayeed Z, Abaab L, El-Othmani M, Pallekonda V, Mihalko W, Saleh KJ. Total Hip Arthroplasty in the Outpatient Setting: What You Need to Know (Part 1). Orthop Clin North Am. 2018;49(1):17-25.

outpatient surgery had lower 30-day complication (3% vs 12%, $P<.001$) and 30-day readmission (3% vs 4%, $P<.001$) rates compared with an inpatient cohort.[15]

Prediction of Success

Of course, appropriate candidate selection and risk stratification can be challenging for any clinician presented with a patient with a range of mild to moderate comorbidities. Several risk stratification algorithms have been described in the literature, with varying efficacy. Two models, the Risk Assessment and Prediction Tool (RAPT) and Outpatient Arthroplasty Risk Assessment (OARA) are the best described and externally validated in the literature.[16] First described in 2003, the RAPT score is a measure that attempts to predict a patient's postoperative rehabilitation needs.[17] The ability of this tool to accurately predict discharge destination after TKA ranges from 62% to 89%, and has had success among patients undergoing primary or revision arthroplasty.[18] One external study found a positive correlation between RAPT score and likelihood of home discharge [OR: 1.59 (CI: 1.43–1.77)]; this correlation was affected by the institution of a multidisciplinary care model.[19] Interestingly, a more recent model from Moore and colleagues outperformed the predictive ability of the RAPT score regardless of whether used in the outpatient or inpatient TKA setting.[13]

The OARA tool was initially described in 2017 and is based on the evaluation of 9 comorbidity categories, each with a proprietary weighted score of specific conditions. In the original description of the OARA score, the metric outperformed both ASA score and Charlson comorbidity index as a predictor for successful outpatient arthroplasty.[20] Further research has shown that both a cutoff score of 60 and 80 have a positive predictive value of more than 90% in predicting successful same-day discharge among patients with TKA and TKA.[20,21] A limitation of the OARA tool seems to be its low negative predictive value and high false-negative rates.[16] Thus, OARA may be useful as a screening instrument to detect patients who are at risk of failing outpatient surgery pathways, but the algorithm may overestimate patient risk. Furthermore, the use of the proprietary weighted system makes application of the results into real-world practice challenging, as the exact effect of variables and influence of practice elements such as analgesia techniques, rehabilitation protocols, and patient education may affect the utility of the scoring system unpredictably. While neither the OARA tool nor RAPT score is faultless, the use of such predictive algorithms is a promising development in the effort to promote appropriate patient selection and prevent unanticipated postoperative hospital admission.

Patient Optimization

Assuming a patient presents for preoperative evaluation with modifiable risk factors, the patient should be medically optimized before surgery. While some exclusion criteria identified in **Box 1** are unmodifiable, a decrease in the severity of certain morbidities could decrease the likelihood of postoperative complications, including the risk of failed outpatient discharge.

Obesity

Obesity is a modifiable risk factor that can impact postsurgical discharge. A large database analysis of complication rates after outpatient TKA or THA found that a BMI more than 35 was an independent risk factor for return to the operating room within 30 days [OR: 1.415 (CI: 1.122–1.784) $P = .003$].[11] In a smaller study of 400 patients undergoing TKA at a single hospital, mean BMI among patients who successfully underwent outpatient surgery was 28.8 kg/m^2, compared with 33.5 kg/m^2 among inpatients.[4] A similar pattern emerges in another NSQIP study, whereby BMI more than 30 was found to be a predictor of a requirement for the length of stay greater than 24 hours, although this effect was more pronounced when BMI was 35 and above.[22] Interestingly, the potential effects of BMI on discharge may also extend to upper extremity arthroplasty. In one analysis of more than 17,000 patients scheduled for shoulder arthroplasty, patients with a BMI greater than 40 were less likely to be in the same-day discharge cohort.[23] Preoperative weight loss should be encouraged in the arthroplasty patient in the presence of obesity. Not only can this facilitate the patient's participation in outpatient surgery but a decrease in the degree of obesity can also decrease the severity and/or impact of associated comorbidities such as hypertension, sleep apnea, and diabetes mellitus.

Anemia

According to one analysis of more than 300,000 patients that underwent a TKA from 2011 to 2018, as many as 10% to 14% of patients may present for TKA with anemia.[24] A recent review of 5384 patients undergoing TJA found that patients with preoperative anemia (defined as Hemoglobin less than 13 g/dL in men and <12 g/dL in women) were 4 times as likely to require a blood transfusion and had approximately a 20% greater length of stay in the hospital.[25] In another study, however, the need for a preoperative blood transfusion was not found to be predictive of an inpatient stay after TKA.[22] Nevertheless, preoperative anemia can have a significant impact on postsurgical risk. For example, in one large NSQIP analysis, preoperative anemia and the need for perioperative blood transfusion were both associated with increased risk of cardiac arrest after TKA.[26] Thus, correction of anemia before TJA can be an issue of patient safety. The use of a blood management program aimed at decreasing the severity of anemia before surgery can be beneficial, and has been associated with decreased length of stay and decreased risk of complications and 90-day readmission.[25,27] Measures to improve anemia may include oral or intravenous iron supplementation, epoetin alfa administration, or preoperative transfusion.[12] Additionally, routine use of tranexamic acid is recommended to decrease the need for perioperative blood transfusion.[28]

Diabetes mellitus

Patients with a history of diabetes mellitus are at increased risk of complications and readmission to the hospital within 30 days after arthroplasty.[11] They are also more likely to require a postoperative stay greater than 24 hours [OR: 1.34 (CI: 1.23–1.47), $P<.0001$].[22] Some evidence suggests that the pathophysiology of the diabetic process can influence the risk of perioperative complications. For example, the presence of insulin-dependent diabetes mellitus before TKA or THA can increase the risk of renal insufficiency compared with non–insulin-dependent diabetes [risk ratio (RR): 2.925 (CI: 1.85–4.626), $P<.001$].[29] The severity of diabetes can also influence the risk of complications after arthroplasty. Historically, a hemoglobin A1C level of more than 8% has been thought to increase the risk of postsurgical infection.[30] However, some studies have suggested that even an A1C between 7% and 8% may be associated with total joint infection.[31] Hence, improvement of glycemic control, potentially to an A1C less than 7%, before surgery should be emphasized during the initial planning stages for arthroplasty.

Albumin

An albumin value less than 3.5 g/dL is commonly used as a marker for mild malnutrition[32][Golladay 2016]. This lower albumin value has been associated with increased risk of infection, readmission, return to the operating room, and complications within 30 days of surgery.[11,33] A recent large NSQIP analysis suggested that hypoalbuminemia may, in fact, be a greater risk factor for negative outcomes than obesity, smoking, or diabetes mellitus.[33] Malnutrition has also been identified as a barrier for same-day discharge after TKA.[4] In one study, instituting a nutritional intervention for arthroplasty patients helped decrease the length of stay and decreased the mean total of all hospital-stay-associated charges [$43,937 (SD $44,164) versus $36,493 (SD $10,494), $P<.001$].[34] Although there is no consensus in the literature regarding when a patient should start a nutritional program before surgery, programs that emphasize high-protein, antiinflammatory diets with appropriate calorie intake are likely beneficial and can also lead to weight loss in the obese patient.

Smoking

While smoking has been associated with higher risk of returning to the operating room within 30 days as well as higher risk of readmission,[11] only limited evidence is available to suggest that smoking is a risk factor for failed outpatient arthroplasty. In one subanalysis of the study of outpatient TKA and THA patients by Sher and colleagues, patients who experienced a severe postdischarge complication or readmission were more likely to be smokers (among other risk factors) (18% vs 13%, $P = .04$).[10] In another large database study, however, smoking was not associated with length of stay.[22] Nevertheless, smoking cessation should be pursued as an objective of preoperative education to decrease the risk of negative outcomes including infection.

Same-Day Versus Next-Day Discharge

With the increasing popularity of outpatient arthroplasty, special consideration should be given to the issue of same-day versus next-day discharge. While same-day surgery may be associated with less utilization of resources and less cost compared with even a one-night stay in a health care facility, some evidence suggests that the latter may be associated with a lesser risk of complications. One study which examined more than 30,000 patients in the NSQIP Medicare database who had undergone THA found that patients who spent one night in the hospital had a decreased risk of reoperation within

30 days (1% vs 3%, $P<.001$) compared with same-day discharge.[15] Another large database study compared outcomes among patients who were discharged same-day, admitted for one night, or were admitted as inpatients after TKA. These authors found that the 30-day risk of any complication was lowest among patients admitted for one night (2%), compared with 8% for same-day discharge patients and 9% for inpatients ($P<.001$).[35] There was, however, no difference in 30-day mortality or 30-day reoperation rates between the 3 groups. While the percentage of patients with pulmonary disease, hypertension, and smoking history was not different among the same-day and next-day discharge cohorts, less patients in the next-day discharge group had a history of diabetes mellitus (16% vs 20%, $P<.001$). Additionally, mean BMI was slightly less in the next-day discharge group (30.8 vs 31.8, $P<.001$). Thus, further studies are needed to compare outcomes among appropriately selected and optimized patients, matched by risk factors and comorbidities, who are discharged the day of surgery versus the following day.

SUMMARY

Although smaller studies suggest that the risk of negative outcomes is equivalent when comparing outpatient and inpatient arthroplasty, larger database analyses suggest that, even when matched for comorbidities, patients undergoing outpatient arthroplasty may be at increased risk of surgical or medical complications. Appropriate patient selection is critical for the success of any outpatient arthroplasty program. Potential exclusion criteria for outpatient TJA may include age greater than 75 years, bleeding disorder, history of deep vein thrombosis, uncontrolled diabetes mellitus, and hypoalbuminemia, among others. Patient optimization before surgery is also warranted. The potential risks of same-day versus next-day discharge have yet to be elicited in a large-scale manner.

CLINICS CARE POINTS

- Criteria that may exclude patients from an outpatient arthroplasty pathway are:
  - Age greater than 75
  - Bleeding disorder/history of deep venous thrombosis
  - Congestive heart failure
  - Significant pulmonary disease
  - Uncontrolled diabetes mellitus (hemoglobin A1C >7)
  - History of chronic pain requiring opioids, substance abuse, or severe uncontrolled postoperative pain
  - Chronic renal disease (Stage 4, glomerular filtration rate <30)
- Algorithmic tools such as RAPT and OARA can be helpful in predicting the risk of postoperative complications or unanticipated admission.
- Certain comorbidities such as obesity, anemia, diabetes mellitus, and hypoalbuminemia should be optimized before surgery to decrease the risk of perioperative complications.
- Even with appropriate patient selection, the risks of perioperative complications may be different among patients discharged on the day of surgery compared with those discharged after an overnight stay.

REFERENCES

1. Singh JA, Yu S, Chen L, et al. Rates of total joint replacement in the United States: future projections to 2020-2040 using the national inpatient sample. J Rheumatol 2019;46(9):1134–40.

2. Rosinsky PJ, Go CC, Bheem R, et al. The cost-effectiveness of outpatient surgery for primary total hip arthroplasty in the United States: a computer-based cost-utility study. Hip Int 2021;31(5):572–81.
3. Keulen MHF, Asselberghs S, Bemelmans YFL, et al. Reasons for unsuccessful same-day discharge following outpatient hip and knee arthroplasty: 5(1/2) years' experience from a single institution. J Arthroplasty 2020;35(9):2327–34.e1.
4. Gillis ME, Dobransky J, Dervin GF. Defining growth potential and barriers to same day discharge total knee arthroplasty. Int Orthop 2019;43(6):1387–93.
5. Buller LT, Hubbard TA, Ziemba-Davis M, et al. Safety of same and next day discharge following revision hip and knee arthroplasty using modern perioperative protocols. J Arthroplasty 2021;36(1):30–6.
6. Rosinsky PJ, Chen SL, Yelton MJ, et al. Outpatient vs. inpatient hip arthroplasty: a matched case-control study on a 90-day complication rate and 2-year patient-reported outcomes. J Orthop Surg Res 2020;15(1):367.
7. Bordoni V, Poggi A, Zaffagnini S, et al. Outpatient total knee arthroplasty leads to a higher number of complications: a meta-analysis. J Orthop Surg Res 2020; 15(1):408.
8. Arshi A, Leong NL, D'Oro A, et al. Outpatient total knee arthroplasty is associated with higher risk of perioperative complications. J Bone Joint Surg Am 2017; 99(23):1978–86.
9. Mai HT, Mukhdomi T, Croxford D, et al. Safety and outcomes of outpatient compared to inpatient total knee arthroplasty: a national retrospective cohort study. Reg Anesth Pain Med 2021;46(1):13–7.
10. Sher A, Keswani A, Yao DH, et al. Predictors of same-day discharge in primary total joint arthroplasty patients and risk factors for post-discharge complications. J Arthroplasty 2017;32(9S):150–6.e1.
11. Courtney PM, Boniello AJ, Berger RA. Complications following outpatient total joint arthroplasty: an analysis of a national database. J Arthroplasty 2017;32(5):1426–30.
12. Sayeed Z, Abaab L, El-Othmani M, et al. Total hip arthroplasty in the outpatient setting: what you need to know (part 1). Orthop Clin North Am 2018;49(1):17–25.
13. Moore MG, Brigati DP, Crijns TJ, et al. Enhanced selection of candidates for same-day and outpatient total knee arthroplasty. J Arthroplasty 2020;35(3):628–32.
14. Toy PC, Fournier MN, Throckmorton TW, et al. Low rates of adverse events following ambulatory outpatient total hip arthroplasty at a free-standing surgery center. J Arthroplasty 2018;33(1):46–50.
15. Greenky MR, Wang W, Ponzio DY, et al. Total hip arthroplasty and the medicare inpatient-only list: an analysis of complications in medicare-aged patients undergoing outpatient surgery. J Arthroplasty 2019;34(6):1250–4.
16. Howie CM, Mears SC, Barnes CL, et al. Readmission, complication, and disposition calculators in total joint arthroplasty: a systemic review. J Arthroplasty 2021; 36(5):1823–31.
17. Oldmeadow LB, McBurney H, Robertson VJ. Predicting risk of extended inpatient rehabilitation after hip or knee arthroplasty. J Arthroplasty 2003;18(6):775–9.
18. Dibra FF, Parvataneni HK, Gray CF, et al. The risk assessment and prediction tool accurately predicts discharge destination after revision hip and knee arthroplasty. J Arthroplasty 2020;35(10):2972–6.
19. Dibra FF, Silverberg AJ, Vasilopoulos T, et al. Arthroplasty care redesign impacts the predictive accuracy of the risk assessment and prediction tool. J Arthroplasty 2019;34(11):2549–54.

20. Meneghini RM, Ziemba-Davis M, Ishmael MK, et al. Safe selection of outpatient joint arthroplasty patients with medical risk stratification: the "outpatient arthroplasty risk assessment score. J Arthroplasty 2017;32(8):2325–31.

21. Ziemba-Davis M, Caccavallo P, Meneghini RM. Outpatient joint arthroplasty-patient selection: update on the outpatient arthroplasty risk assessment score. J Arthroplasty 2019;34(7S):S40–3.

22. Johnson DJ, Castle JP, Hartwell MJ, et al. Risk factors for greater than 24-hour length of stay after primary total knee arthroplasty. J Arthroplasty 2020;35(3): 633–7.

23. Burton BN, Finneran JJ, Angerstein A, et al. Demographic and clinical factors associated with same-day discharge and unplanned readmission following shoulder arthroplasty: a retrospective cohort study. Korean J Anesthesiol 2021; 74(1):30–7.

24. Warren JA, McLaughlin JP, Molloy RM, et al. Blood management in total knee arthroplasty: a nationwide analysis from 2011 to 2018. J Knee Surg 2020. https://doi.org/10.1055/s-0040-1721414.

25. Bailey A, Eisen I, Palmer A, et al. Preoperative anemia in primary arthroplasty patients-prevalence, influence on outcome, and the effect of treatment. J Arthroplasty 2021;36(7):2281–9.

26. Kataria R, Iniguez R, Foy M, et al. Preoperative risk factors for postoperative cardiac arrest following primary total hip and knee arthroplasty: A large database study. J Clin Orthop Trauma 2021;16:244–8.

27. Rogers BA, Cowie A, Alcock C, et al. Identification and treatment of anaemia in patients awaiting hip replacement. Ann R Coll Surg Engl 2008;90(6):504–7.

28. Poeran J, Chan JJ, Zubizarreta N, et al. Safety of tranexamic acid in hip and knee arthroplasty in high-risk patients. Anesthesiology 2021;135(1):57–68.

29. Wu LM, Si HB, Li MY, et al. Insulin dependence increases the risk of complications and death in total joint arthroplasty: a systematic review and meta-(regression) analysis. Orthop Surg 2021;13(3):719–33.

30. Han HS, Kang SB. Relations between long-term glycemic control and postoperative wound and infectious complications after total knee arthroplasty in type 2 diabetics. Clin Orthop Surg 2013;5(2):118–23.

31. Cancienne JM, Werner BC, Browne JA. Is there a threshold value of hemoglobin a1c that predicts risk of infection following primary total hip arthroplasty? J Arthroplasty 2017;32(9S):S236–40.

32. Golladay GJ, Satpathy J, Jiranek WA. Patient optimization-strategies that work: malnutrition. J Arthroplasty 2016;31(8):1631–4.

33. Johnson NR, Statz JM, Odum SM, et al. Failure to optimize before total knee arthroplasty: which modifiable risk factor is the most dangerous? J Arthroplasty 2021;36(7):2452–7.

34. Schroer WC, LeMarr AR, Mills K, et al. 2019 Chitranjan S. Ranawat Award: Elective joint arthroplasty outcomes improve in malnourished patients with nutritional intervention: a prospective population analysis demonstrates a modifiable risk factor. Bone Joint J 2019;101-B(7_Supple_C):17–21.

35. Courtney PM, Froimson MI, Meneghini RM, et al. Can Total Knee Arthroplasty Be Performed Safely as an Outpatient in the Medicare Population? J Arthroplasty 2018;33(7S):S28–31.

Regional Anesthesia in the Elite Athlete

Patrick Meyer, MD*, Kristopher Schroeder, MD

KEYWORDS

- Athlete • Regional anesthesia • Nerve block • Nerve injury • Analgesia • Consent

KEY POINTS

- Regional anesthesia is safe and the risk of perioperative nerve injury is incredibly low, but consideration of even minor or temporary nerve dysfunction and the implications for an elite athlete must be considered.
- The risks, benefits, and alternatives to regional anesthesia interventions should be discussed in-depth in the context of each athlete's unique circumstance.
- The risks of opioid analgesics must be discussed with patients and a patient's personal pain history and opioid experience should be considered when planning a perioperative analgesic regimen.
- If regional anesthesia is performed, strategies to decrease the risk of injury should be used
- Documentation of the consent discussion and the procedure details should be thorough to serve as a record of the care provided.

INTRODUCTION

In the United States and throughout the world, professional athletes are revered and their injuries and medical treatment frequently constitute headline news. The accomplishments of these athletes serve as a source of civic pride and the success of a team or a charismatic athlete may result in billions of dollars in revenue for local communities. Unfortunately, the very nature of an athlete's profession exposes them to an elevated risk of injury that often involves the musculoskeletal system. These injuries can be career defining, and the management of their injury and associated pain is of crucial importance to an elite athlete.

When considering the postoperative analgesic management of accomplished athletes, there is a multitude of potentially competing concerns that must be considered by the patient, anesthesiologist, and surgeon. For example, a patient's individual pain tolerance and history of opioid use should be considered and this may influence the analgesic plan. For many of these athletes, there may be a high degree of opioid

Department of Anesthesiology, University of Wisconsin, 600 Highland Avenue, Madison, WI 53792, USA
* Corresponding author.
E-mail address: psmeyer@wisc.edu

Clin Sports Med 41 (2022) 291–302
https://doi.org/10.1016/j.csm.2021.11.008
0278-5919/22/© 2021 Elsevier Inc. All rights reserved.

consumption and potential for the development of tolerance. In fact, a recent study found that high school athletes had a lifetime opioid use rate of 28% to 46% and that 52% of National Football League players had required opioid administration at some point during their career.[1] The location of the injury and the ability to administer a regional anesthesia technique that provides an isolated sensory block or greatly facilitates the ability to participate in physical rehabilitation may "tip the scales" toward the utilization of these techniques. On the other hand, these high-functioning athletes may also be more likely to be detrimentally impacted by relatively minor decreases in strength or sensation that could result from a block-related nerve injury and this should be considered and discussed with these patients in depth.

What follows is a detailed discussion of some of the considerations associated with the provision of perioperative analgesia for elite athletes and those that derive significant fulfillment from participation in athletic events. While the intent of this article is to focus on the unique situation encountered in the analgesic and perioperative care of athletes, many of the concepts could be used when caring for other high-performing individuals (ie, singers requiring mechanical ventilation; a surgeon requiring fine dexterity for procedures).

DEFINING THE RISKS

Professional athletes are required to push their body to the extremes of physical conditioning to perform at their peak, which unfortunately predisposes them to injury. Injury limits an athlete's ability to perform and is a threat to their livelihood. Recovery from an injury that requires surgical intervention exposes athletes to surgical and anesthetic risks that are magnified by a narrow tolerance for postoperative functional decline or prolonged recovery. The risk of postoperative neurologic symptoms (PONS) following regional anesthesia/analgesia may adversely impact an athlete's recovery following injury and surgical intervention. Neurologic injuries following peripheral nerve blockade are rare, with estimates ranging from 2.4 to 4 per 10,000 blocks.[2–7] Nerve injury may be secondary to needle trauma, pressure injury from local anesthetic injection or hematoma formation, ischemia, or via direct effects from perineural administration of local anesthetic and/or adjuvant medications.[8,9] These risks are further altered by the anatomic location of a proposed regional anesthetic procedure[7] and the planned surgical intervention.[10] PONS are also greatly influenced by patient-specific characteristics.[11,12]

Isolating the risk of neurologic dysfunction associated with regional nerve blocks from the risks associated with surgery, positioning, tourniquet use, or other insults can be challenging. In fact, a prospective case series that evaluated over 7000 peripheral nerve blocks found that a diagnosis of a PONS was 9 times more likely to be secondary to a non-nerve block cause than a result of the nerve block itself.[2] A large retrospective study evaluating nerve injury found that peripheral nerve block administration was not an independent risk factor for perioperative nerve injury, although general and epidural anesthesia were.[13] Other studies have shown no association between peripheral nerve blockade and perioperative nerve injury following total knee arthroplasty,[14] total hip arthroplasty,[15] and total shoulder arthroplasty.[16] Nonetheless, the risk of nerve dysfunction from a nerve block is not zero and the risk of subclinical dysfunction that goes undetected in the general population but may manifest in an elite athlete must be considered.

Of particular concern to an athlete is the risk that a nerve block could contribute to decreased strength or a delay in function that slows or prevents return to sport. The impact of perioperative regional anesthesia on functional recovery following ACL reconstruction has been extensively researched. A 2015 cohort study evaluated iso-kinetic muscle strength at 6 months following ACL reconstruction surgery in patients who either received or did not receive an analgesic femoral nerve block (FNB).[17] Despite similar graft types, those who received an FNB had significantly decreased isokinetic strength deficits with knee extension and flexion 6 months after surgery compared with those who did not receive a block. Additionally, those who did not receive a FNB were four times more likely to be cleared for return to sport at 6 months. In another retrospective study, Everhart and colleagues reported a decrease in isoki-netic strength and increased risk of ACL graft rupture within the first year after surgery when a FNB was used for perioperative analgesia for ACL repair.[18] A 2017 randomized controlled trial (RCT) reported decreased quadriceps strength in those patients who received a perioperative FNB at 6 weeks but this did not persist at 6 months.[19] Ath-letes understandingly may be concerned by any procedure potentially accompanied by a risk of delayed or decreased function, delayed return to sport or increased risk of career-defining reinjury. Subsequent studies, including an RCT comparing quadri-ceps strength in patients receiving either a FNB or injection of local anesthetic at the surgery site at a later time-point (9 months), found no difference between groups,[20] while a recent cohort study reported knee flexor strength deficits in those who received a sciatic nerve block at the time of return to sport (5–7 months) but found no difference in knee extensor strength in those who received a FNB compared with those who did not.[21] Efforts to address the possibility of decreased functional re-covery secondary to motor nerve involvement with the administration of a FNB led to increased interest in the perioperative provision of an adductor canal block (ACB) for ACL reconstruction surgery. Early preoperative strength testing after nerve blockade did indeed find a preservation of quadricep strength in the ACB compared with the FNB,[22] but further studies have found conflicting results at later time points of assess-ment.[23,24] These studies highlight both the concern for nerve-block related neurologic dysfunction and the difficulty in clearly defining risks for patients given the numerous patient-specific and environmental influences that affect an athlete's recovery following injury and surgery. These risks must be balanced against the risks of alter-native anesthetic and analgesic treatment modalities, which are also difficult to quan-tify. The consequences for an athlete unable to rehabilitate to their prior form following a musculoskeletal injury can be significant including the loss of playing time, scholar-ship, salary, and endorsements—whether secondary to the injury itself, the surgery or anesthesia required, or the analgesic modality used to control perioperative pain.

Physicians caring for elite athletes may be concerned about the medical-legal risks of performing regional anesthetic techniques in this patient population. The review of closed-claims databases suggests a relatively high percentage of anesthesia-related claims result from peripheral and neuraxial analgesic block complications.[25] High pro-file cases of professional athletes seeking financial remuneration for damages claimed to be a result of surgical and anesthetic procedures may appropriately provoke appre-hension when planning a regional anesthesia procedure in a high-level athlete.[26] These considerations must be balanced with the knowledge that permanent nerve injury following peripheral nerve blocks is exceptionally rare in the general population and the known and serious risks of alternative anesthetic and analgesic treatment op-tions. Regional anesthesia and peripheral nerve blocks have been associated with decreased postanesthesia care unit use, decreased nausea, decreased postoperative pain,[27] and a decreased risk of persistent postoperative pain.[28] It is the task of the anesthesiologist to collaborate with the athlete in the preoperative arena and, through shared decision making, develop an anesthetic and perioperative pain management plan that addresses the patient's concerns and appropriately informs the patient of the risks associated with the available options. In addition, efforts should be made to minimize these risks and optimize operating conditions for the surgical team. If regional anesthesia is selected, strategies to improve safety and minimize the risks associated with the procedure should be undertaken.

STRATEGIES THAT MAY INCREASE SAFETY

Many of the strategies used by anesthesiologists to decrease the risks of regional anesthesia in athletes are tactics that can be applied to all patients. In an elite athlete, minimizing the occurrence and magnitude of neuromuscular dysfunction can be vital to ensuring a return to sport at a high level of performance.

Ultrasound Guidance

The use of ultrasound guidance in regional anesthesia has grown tremendously over the last several decades. The rapid advancements in ultrasound technology have allowed for increasing resolution and more mobile platforms that have resulted in widespread adoption in the field. Ultrasound has pushed the boundaries of regional anesthesia, with the ever-increasing adoption of fascial plane blocks and neuraxial applications that have been made possible with these technologic improvements. Ultrasound allows for the identification of anatomic structures and visualization of the needle path throughout the procedure. The ability to clearly identify the nerve target and needle tip location, blood vessels in the path of the needle, and visualize local anesthetic spread is possible mechanisms for the reported increased safety profiles associated with the use of ultrasound guidance for the provision of regional anesthesia. Indeed, a recent meta-analysis demonstrated that ultrasound guidance has been shown to reduce the incidence and intensity of hemidiaphragmatic paresis with interscalene blocks, reduce the incidence of pneumothorax with supraclavicular blocks, and reduce the incidence of local anesthetic systemic toxicity (LAST) up to 65%.[29] Nonetheless, the same meta-analysis concluded that evidence has continued to show that ultrasound guidance does not meaningfully affect the incidence of peripheral nerve injury associated with regional anesthesia. Intrafascicular injections are felt to carry the highest risk of nerve injury. The ability to reliably differentiate an intrafascicular injection from an extrafascicular injection with ultrasound imaging may require continued technologic improvements in ultrasound resolution. This differentiation is also dependent on patient-specific factors affecting image acquisition (depth of target) and the ability of the user to accurately differentiate injectate spread.

There are several well-accepted techniques that should be used to improve the safety of ultrasound-guided regional techniques. Before any nerve block, a preprocedure scan that uses color Doppler can help identify vascular structures within the planned needle trajectory and allow for reassessment to minimize vessel disruption, hematoma development, and potentially limit risk for intravascular injection and LAST.[30] In addition, maintaining clear visualization of the entire needle throughout the approach to the target is crucial. Using a shallow angle, optimizing tilt and rotation of the probe, and considering the use of echogenic needles can improve needle visualization. Using hydrodissection can further define needle-tip location and may be used to create a space in which to safely advance the needle while avoiding needle placement needlessly close to a nerve target. Local anesthetic deposition should be carefully monitored with ultrasound, as tissue spread should minimize the risk of direct intravascular injection, verify appropriate spread around the target and exclude, as best as possible, intraneural and intramuscular injection.

Nerve Stimulation

The use of a nerve stimulator may help to facilitate the appropriate positioning of the needle tip near the nerve, confirm that structure is indeed a nerve, and may help to avoid intraneural injections. Peripheral nerve stimulation relies on the fact that smaller current intensities are required to elicit a sensory or motor response as the needle tip is moved closer to the corresponding nerve. With the widespread use of ultrasound guidance, peripheral nerve stimulation continues to retain value as a safety adjunct and may assist in the identification/localization of difficult to visualize nerves or plexuses, enhance block success and minimize the intraneural injection of local anesthetics. Research has demonstrated that a motor response with a delivered current amplitude of 0.2 mA or less reliably indicates intraneural needle placement.[31,32] However, stimulation currents of more than 0.2 mA and no more than 0.5 mA could not rule out intraneural needle positioning.[31] These findings suggest that eliciting a motor response at a current intensity of less than 0.5 mA likely represents intraneural or close needle-nerve contact and warrants close attention to injectate spread patterns or needle repositioning before local anesthetic injection. It is important to note that the absence of a motor response to nerve stimulation does not exclude intraneural needle placement and repeated attempts to elicit motor stimulation may lead to unnecessary redirection and an increased risk of nerve injury.[33] With the widespread availability of high-resolution ultrasound technology, a prudent approach to safely administering nerve blocks may use a dual-endpoint technique that features both ultrasound guidance to facilitate needle placement and peripheral nerve stimulation to exclude motor responses at less than 0.2 mA before injection to minimize the risk of intraneural injection and peripheral nerve injury.

Injection Pressure Monitoring

A further mechanism designed to reduce the incidence or severity of nerve injury associated with peripheral nerve blockade is through monitoring the pressure associated with local anesthetic injection. Pressure manometers can be used during nerve block procedures to guide injection. High injection pressure may indicate intraneural needle placement that may predispose an individual to increased risk of nerve injury. Histologic evaluation of nerves reveals marked abnormalities associated with intraneural injections of ropivacaine, with milder damage seen with extrafascicular injection.[34] Several animal studies have been conducted that demonstrate persistent neurologic deficits associated with high injection pressure.[8,35] In humans, Gadsden and colleagues demonstrated that needle tip placement 1 mm away from the nerve root during an interscalene block consistently resulted in opening injection pressures of less than 15 psi. In instances of needle-nerve contact, opening injection pressures were greater than 15 psi in 35 of 36 injections.[36] Similarly, an opening injection pressure of greater than 15 psi was associated with a block needle tip position indenting the epineurium of the femoral nerve in 90% of the assessments, with opening pressures of less than 15 psi in all cases whereby the needle was at least 1 mm away from the nerve.[37] These studies suggest that monitoring injection pressure and repositioning the needle tip to achieve an opening injection pressure of less than 15 psi may provide additional safety mechanisms to prevent intraneural injection. Several disposable manometer devices are commercially available at a relatively low cost per use.

Level of Sedation

Limiting sedation during the procedure may be helpful in ensuring that patients are able to provide feedback regarding any elicited paresthesia or pain with injection or needle advancement. Nerve injury has been documented to occur with and without pain or paresthesia, but pain and/or paresthesia with injection would suggest intraneural injection and certainly prompt needle repositioning, potentially offering an additional safety mechanism against injury. The availability of this feedback needs to be balanced with the potential risks associated with a patient that is highly anxious or otherwise unable to remain motionless throughout the procedure.

For a variety of reasons, regional anesthesia is often performed before the induction of anesthesia and surgical manipulation. The provision of this preemptive analgesia may offer a variety of analgesic benefits including limiting the development of opioid-induced hyperalgesia, minimizing anesthetic requirements, and improving the postoperative condition and recovery efficiency of surgical patients. One risk of providing regional anesthesia in the preoperative arena to all patients is the potential for overutilization in patients who may have recovered without the requirement of a PNB, thus exposing them to the inherent risks of regional. By postoperatively documenting normal sensory and motor examination before performing regional anesthesia, there may be greater ability to more judiciously administer regional anesthesia and limit liability should an adverse event occur. However, it is important to consider that performing regional anesthesia following surgery does have potential implications that should be considered. For example, following a general anesthetic, these patients may be limited in their ability to report significant pain associated with the regional anesthesia procedure and local anesthetic injection. In addition, performing postoperative blocks may impose positioning limitations or bandaging may limit approach options. The ability to use a nerve stimulator as a safety adjunct may be negated in a patient experiencing significant postoperative pain. Finally, patients are likely to have higher anesthetic requirements and greater opioid needs if blocks are not performed preoperatively, thus negating some of the benefits of regional techniques.

The American Society of Regional Anesthesia and Pain Medicine (ASRA) practice advisory on neurologic complications has shared expert opinion regarding the provision of peripheral nerve blocks and neuraxial procedure on anesthetized or heavily-sedated patients.[38] They recommend that neuraxial procedures and peripheral nerve blockade should not be routinely performed in most adults during general anesthesia or heavy sedation. They acknowledge that the decision is controversial, complicated, and must be made in the absence of traditional forms of evidence-based medicine.

Other Considerations

In some cases whereby surgical anesthesia is not required, the use of lower concentration local anesthetics for analgesia may provide an increased safety margin. All local anesthetics are known to be neurotoxic and the level of toxicity correlates with increasing concentration and duration of exposure.[39,40] Using a lower concentration of local anesthetic for analgesic blocks may therefore limit toxicity while still providing sufficient analgesia. The adjuvant epinephrine is often used as a marker for intravascular injection. However, epinephrine induces vasoconstriction that extends the exposure of nerves to local anesthetics and decreases blood flow to the nerve which may expose the nerves to greater risk of ischemia.[41] This risk should be balanced with the risk of undetected intravascular injection and potential development of LAST. The risks of epinephrine are especially critical to consider in those who already have existing nerve injury or are at risk of undetected nerve damage (ie, uncontrolled diabetes), or in those who may be exposed to multiple additional insults perioperatively (ie, ischemia secondary to tourniquet use). Limiting additional nerve toxicity in these situations may help avoid or lessen the risk of nerve injury secondary to the "double crush" phenomenon.[42]

For many surgical procedures, there are a variety of regional anesthesia options that might accomplish successful analgesia but limit the risks of the regional intervention. For example, targeting a purely sensory nerve (ie, saphenous) for lower extremity surgery may offer significant benefits relative to targeting a nerve that has both sensory and motor components. As another example, the suprascapular nerve provides significant sensory innervation to the shoulder and may present an improved safety profile relative to an interscalene block for shoulder surgery given the location distant from the brachial plexus roots and phrenic nerve. Finally, using regional anesthesia techniques with a well-defined and bony backstop may introduce a level of safety versus techniques that require needle advancement toward soft-tissue or pleural endpoints. For example, in athletes with rib fractures, a serratus or erector spinae plane block may represent a safer alternative versus an intercostal nerve block.

Finally, the provision of regional anesthesia in the high-functioning/high-profile athlete is not something that should be managed by a novice or someone who dabbles in regional anesthesia. These procedures are best reserved for anesthesiologists with extensive experience or training in the provision of advanced regional anesthesia techniques.

Ideally, the implementation of these strategies piece together a plan that represents the best or most risk-avoidant approach (**Fig. 1**). Whatever techniques are implemented, thorough documentation should be completed and significant time should be dedicated to explaining the risks, benefits, and alternatives to regional procedures in athletes.

Consent Considerations

There are 3 basic elements of informed consent that are universal and required for all patients—threshold elements, information elements, and consent elements[43] (**Fig. 2**). The threshold elements represent competence and voluntariness. Voluntariness requires a patient to be free from coercion and permission to proceed with an intervention is given freely. For the elite athlete, it is important to recognize the influence that

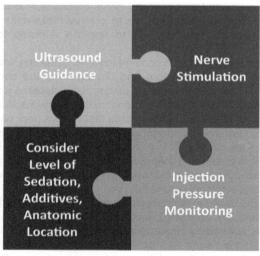

Fig. 1. Piecing together a safe regional anesthesia plan.

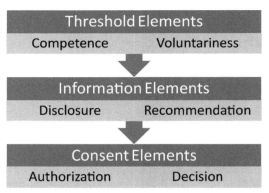

Fig. 2. Elements of informed consent.

agents, coaches, trainers, and other team personnel might have on a patient's decision to proceed with a regional anesthetic intervention. While these people may provide valuable guidance, it is important the patient is able to make the best decision for themselves. The information disclosed during the consent process should detail the risks, benefits, and alternatives to a proposed procedure and understanding of these concepts should be ensured. The legal obligation for the materiality of the consent usually requires the information to meet the accepted professional practice standard of care or the reasonable person standard, which is the information a hypothetical person would want to know to make an informed decision.[44] The information disclosed regarding a specific procedure should be tailored to the individual patient. For example, the extremely low risk of permanent nerve injury or the risk of a temporary decrease in muscle function that may be acceptable to a nonathlete given some of the short-term benefits of the intervention may not be acceptable for an elite athlete given the consequences these rare outcomes may have for their career. Unfortunately, these standards are often not met. In a recent survey of regional anesthesiologists at academic institutions, nearly 40% did not disclose the risk of long-term nerve injury to patients undergoing central or peripheral nerve blockade.[45] It is incumbent on the anesthesiologist caring for these patients to convey these risks to the patient in a manner that they can understand and to reach a decision for which they are comfortable.

The final component of informed consent involves obtaining written or verbal consent or authorization for a procedure and documenting the consent process that took place. Documentation of the consent discussion in detail as well as any questions raised by the athlete is vitally important to ensure that there is a record of this process. Multiple published studies have demonstrated that there is poor patient recall of anesthesia consent discussions and therefore, documentation ensures that this process and the discussion are codified.[46,47] In addition, alterations to an institution's normal practice that were implemented following a discussion with the patient athlete (as-needed postoperative regional anesthesia, foregoing regional anesthesia, decreased local anesthetic concentration, etc.) should be clearly documented before the procedure. The manner and timing in which regional anesthesia is presented to patients vary without a clear champion regarding the presentation method. In an ideal scenario, any proposed regional anesthesia procedure would be discussed with athletes well in advance of their planned surgical procedure to facilitate their ability to research the proposed intervention and formulate questions. In-person discussions with an anesthesiologist help build rapport and ensure that an individual anesthesiologist's experience and comfort with a proposed treatment regimen can be discussed with an individual patient. However, this method may fail if individual providers are uneducated about the risk associated with the proposed procedures or if there is inadequate time to devote to this important process. Standardized print or audio–visual materials may help to ensure that patients receive risk information but they fail to ensure that this information is viewed or understandable to the patient. A combination of verbal and written consent may offer benefits to each and may improve retention of the consent itself.[48] Regardless of the method used, anesthesiologists have both a legal and an ethical obligation to the patient to achieve informed consent before any regional intervention.

ALTERNATIVES TO REGIONAL ANESTHESIA

While regional anesthesia represents the "gold standard" for perioperative analgesia in the setting of many orthopedic procedures, there may be some cases whereby the anticipated benefits are outweighed by the magnitude of potential risks. In these situations, consideration should be given to the administration of alternative analgesic techniques less likely to impact nerve function. Maximizing the administration of multimodal agents such as ketamine, magnesium, intravenous lidocaine, NSAIDS, acetaminophen, and alpha-2 agonists may achieve significant analgesic benefits and, in some cases, obviate the need for regional anesthesia. Ensuring that patients are educated and prepared for surgery, informed and appropriately counseled about the expectations of pain, and provided an opportunity to practice alternative, nonpharmacologic techniques such as mindfulness or distraction techniques are all important in the peri-operative process.

SUMMARY

Elite athletes are exposed to an elevated risk of musculoskeletal injury. These injuries, and the risks associated with their treatment and rehabilitation, may constitute a significant threat to an athlete's livelihood. Further, their careers require a return to elite performance functioning in an efficient manner that provides little room for even minor or temporary changes to neuromuscular function. In addition, pain control could prove challenging in the event of preoperative analgesic use, just as with any other surgical patient. Regional anesthesia has numerous perioperative benefits. However, the risks of these interventions must be thoroughly understood and considered in the context of an athlete's often low tolerance for complications. The risks of these procedures should be clearly explained and alternatives discussed to allow the athlete to participate in the development of an analgesic care plan that best balances these considerations for their unique situation. The risks of regional anesthesia alternatives (ie, opioids, general anesthesia) must be thoroughly discussed and balanced against the risks of regional anesthesia. If regional anesthesia is used, overlapping strategies to cumulatively decrease the risks associated with the procedures should be used and documentation should be thorough to serve as a record for this detailed process. Through this thoughtful approach, clinicians can provide the most appropriate care for each athlete and partner with them on their journey back to their prior form.

DISCLOSURE

The authors have nothing to disclose.

CLINICS CARE POINTS

- Regional anesthesia is safe and the risk of perioperative nerve injury is incredibly low, but consideration of even minor or temporary nerve dysfunction and the implications for an elite athlete must be considered

- The risks, benefits, and alternatives to regional anesthesia interventions should be discussed in-depth in the context of each athlete's unique circumstance

- The risks of opioid analgesics must be discussed with patients and a patient's personal pain history and opioid experience should be considered when planning a perioperative analgesic regimen

- If regional anesthesia is performed, strategies to decrease the risk of injury should be used

- Documentation of the consent discussion and the procedure details should be thorough to serve as a record of the care provided

REFERENCES

1. Ekhtiari S, Yusuf I, AlMakadma Y, et al. Opioid use in athletes: a systematic review. Sports Health 2020;12(6):534–9.
2. Barrington MJ, Watts SA, Gledhill SR, et al. Preliminary results of the Australasian Regional Anaesthesia Collaboration: a prospective audit of more than 7000 peripheral nerve and plexus blocks for neurologic and other complications. Reg Anesth Pain Med 2009;34(6):534–41.
3. Auroy Y, Benhamou D, Bargues L, et al. Major complications of regional anesthesia in France: The SOS Regional Anesthesia Hotline Service. Anesthesiology 2002;97(5):1274–80.
4. Fredrickson MJ, Kilfoyle DH. Neurological complication analysis of 1000 ultrasound guided peripheral nerve blocks for elective orthopaedic surgery: a prospective study. Anaesthesia 2009;64(8):836–44.
5. Orebaugh SL, Kentor ML, Williams BA. Adverse outcomes associated with nerve stimulator-guided and ultrasound-guided peripheral nerve blocks by supervised trainees: update of a single-site database. Reg Anesth Pain Med 2012;37(6):577–82.
6. Orebaugh SL, Williams BA, Vallejo M, et al. Adverse outcomes associated with stimulator-based peripheral nerve blocks with versus without ultrasound visualization. Reg Anesth Pain Med 2009;34(3):251–5.
7. Sites BD, Taenzer AH, Herrick MD, et al. Incidence of local anesthetic systemic toxicity and postoperative neurologic symptoms associated with 12,668 ultrasound-guided nerve blocks: an analysis from a prospective clinical registry. Reg Anesth Pain Med 2012;37(5):478–82.
8. Hadzic A, Dilberovic F, Shah S, et al. Combination of intraneural injection and high injection pressure leads to fascicular injury and neurologic deficits in dogs. Reg Anesth Pain Med 2004;29(5):417–23.
9. Borgeat A, Blumenthal S. Nerve injury and regional anaesthesia. Curr Opin Anaesthesiol 2004;17(5):417–21.
10. Rodeo SA, Forster RA, Weiland AJ. Neurological complications due to arthroscopy. J Bone Joint Surg Am 1993;75(6):917–26.
11. Hebl JR. Peripheral nerve injury. In: Neal JM, Rathmell JP, editors. Complications in regional anesthesia and pain medicine. 2ND edition. Philadelphia: Wolters Kluwer Health/Lippincott Williams & Wilkins; 2013. p. 150-169.

12. Horlocker TT, O'Driscoll SW, Dinapoli RP. Recurring brachial plexus neuropathy in a diabetic patient after shoulder surgery and continuous interscalene block. Anesth Analg 2000;91(3):688–90.

13. Welch MB, Brummett CM, Welch TD, et al. Perioperative peripheral nerve injuries: a retrospective study of 380,680 cases during a 10-year period at a single institution. Anesthesiology 2009;111(3):490–7.

14. Jacob AK, Mantilla CB, Sviggum HP, et al. Perioperative nerve injury after total knee arthroplasty: regional anesthesia risk during a 20-year cohort study. Anesthesiology 2011;114(2):311–7.

15. Jacob AK, Mantilla CB, Sviggum HP, et al. Perioperative nerve injury after total hip arthroplasty: regional anesthesia risk during a 20-year cohort study. Anesthesiology 2011;115(6):1172–8.

16. Sviggum HP, Jacob AK, Mantilla CB, et al. Perioperative nerve injury after total shoulder arthroplasty: assessment of risk after regional anesthesia. Reg Anesth Pain Med 2012;37(5):490–4.

17. Luo TD, Ashraf A, Dahm DL, et al. Femoral nerve block is associated with persistent strength deficits at 6 months after anterior cruciate ligament reconstruction in pediatric and adolescent patients. Am J Sports Med 2015;43(2):331–6.

18. Everhart JS, Hughes L, Abouljoud MM, et al. Femoral nerve block at time of ACL reconstruction causes lasting quadriceps strength deficits and may increase short-term risk of re-injury. Knee Surg Sports Traumatol Arthrosc 2020;28(6):1894–900.

19. Magnussen RA, Pottkotter K, Stasi SD, et al. Femoral Nerve Block after Anterior Cruciate Ligament Reconstruction. J Knee Surg 2017;30(4):323–8.

20. Okoroha KR, Khalil L, Jung EK, et al. Single-shot femoral nerve block does not cause long-term strength and functional deficits following anterior cruciate ligament reconstruction. Arthroscopy 2018;34(1):205–12.

21. Kew ME, Bodkin SG, Diduch DR, et al. The Influence of Perioperative Nerve Block on Strength and Functional Return to Sports After Anterior Cruciate Ligament Reconstruction. Am J Sports Med 2020;48(7):1689–95.

22. Abdallah FW, Whelan DB, Chan VW, et al. Adductor canal block provides noninferior analgesia and superior quadriceps strength compared with femoral nerve block in anterior cruciate ligament reconstruction. Anesthesiology 2016;124(5):1053–64.

23. Runner RP, Boden SA, Godfrey WS, et al. Quadriceps strength deficits after a femoral nerve block versus adductor canal block for anterior cruciate ligament reconstruction: a prospective, single-blinded, randomized trial. Orthop J Sports Med 2018;6(9). 2325967118797990.

24. Christensen JE, Taylor NE, Hetzel SJ, et al. Isokinetic Strength Deficit 6 Months After Adductor Canal Blockade for Anterior Cruciate Ligament Reconstruction. Orthop J Sports Med 2017;5(11). 2325967117736249.

25. Peng PW, Smedstad KG. Litigation in Canada against anesthesiologists practicing regional anesthesia. A review of closed claims. Can J Anaesth 2000;47(2):105–12.

26. McCann M. Diving Into Sharrif Floyd's $180M suit vs. Dr. Andrews. Sports Illustrated. Available at: https://www.si.com/nfl/2018/11/07/minnesota-vikings-sharrif-floyds-180-million-lawsuit-against-dr-james-andrews. Accessed June 28, 2021.

27. Liu SS, Strodtbeck WM, Richman JM, et al. A comparison of regional versus general anesthesia for ambulatory anesthesia: a meta-analysis of randomized controlled trials. Anesth Analg 2005;101(6):1634–42.

28. Levene JL, Weinstein EJ, Cohen MS, et al. Local anesthetics and regional anesthesia versus conventional analgesia for preventing persistent postoperative pain

in adults and children: A Cochrane systematic review and meta-analysis update. J Clin Anesth 2019;55:116–27.

29. Neal JM. Ultrasound-Guided Regional Anesthesia and Patient Safety: Update of an Evidence-Based Analysis. Reg Anesth Pain Med 2016;41(2):195–204.

30. Manickam BP, Perlas A, Chan VWS, et al. The role of a preprocedure systematic sonographic survey in ultrasound-guided regional anesthesia. Reg Anesth Pain Med 2008;33(6):566–70.

31. Bigeleisen PE, Moayeri N, Groen GJ. Extraneural versus intraneural stimulation thresholds during ultrasound-guided supraclavicular block. Anesthesiology 2009;110(6):1235–43.

32. Tsai TP, Vuckovic I, Dilberovic F, et al. Intensity of the stimulating current may not be a reliable indicator of intraneural needle placement. Reg Anesth Pain Med 2008;33(3):207–10.

33. Robards C, Hadzic A, Somasundaram L, et al. Intraneural injection with low-current stimulation during popliteal sciatic nerve block. Anesth Analg 2009;109(2):673–7.

34. Whitlock EL, Brenner MJ, Fox IK, et al. Ropivacaine-induced peripheral nerve injection injury in the rodent model. Anesth Analg 2010;111(1):214–20.

35. Kapur E, Vuckovic I, Dilberovic F, et al. Neurologic and histologic outcome after intraneural injections of lidocaine in canine sciatic nerves. Acta Anaesthesiol Scand 2007;51(1):101–7.

36. Gadsden JC, Choi JJ, Lin E, et al. Opening injection pressure consistently detects needle-nerve contact during ultrasound-guided interscalene brachial plexus block. Anesthesiology 2014;120(5):1246–53.

37. Gadsden J, Latmore M, Levine DM, et al. High Opening Injection Pressure Is Associated With Needle-Nerve and Needle-Fascia Contact During Femoral Nerve Block. Reg Anesth Pain Med 2016;41(1):50–5.

38. Bernards CM, Hadzic A, Suresh S, et al. Regional anesthesia in anesthetized or heavily sedated patients. Reg Anesth Pain Med 2008;33(5):449–60.

39. Yang S, Abrahams MS, Hurn PD, et al. Local anesthetic Schwann cell toxicity is time and concentration dependent. Reg Anesth Pain Med 2011;36(5):444–51.

40. Werdehausen R, Fazeli S, Braun S, et al. Apoptosis induction by different local anaesthetics in a neuroblastoma cell line. Br J Anaesth 2009;103(5):711–8.

41. Hogan QH. Pathophysiology of peripheral nerve injury during regional anesthesia. Reg Anesth Pain Med 2008;33(5):435–41.

42. Upton AR, McComas AJ. The double crush in nerve entrapment syndromes. Lancet 1973;2(7825):359–62.

43. Beauchamp TL, Childress JF. Principles of biomedical ethics. OUP USA; 2013. Available at: https://books.google.com/books?id=I9VIMQEACAAJ.

44. Waisel DB, Truog RD. Informed consent. Anesthesiology 1997;87(4):968–78.

45. Brull R, McCartney CJL, Chan VWS, et al. Disclosure of risks associated with regional anesthesia: a survey of academic regional anesthesiologists. Reg Anesth Pain Med 2007;32(1):7–11.

46. Tait AR, Voepel-Lewis T, Gauger V. Parental recall of anesthesia information: informing the practice of informed consent. Anesth Analg 2011;112(4):918–23.

47. Zarnegar R, Brown MRD, Henley M, et al. Patient perceptions and recall of consent for regional anaesthesia compared with consent for surgery. J R Soc Med 2015;108(11):451–6.

48. Gerancher JC, Grice SC, Dewan DM, et al. An evaluation of informed consent prior to epidural analgesia for labor and delivery. Int J Obstet Anesth 2000;9(3):168–73.

Local Anesthetics, Local Anesthetic Systemic Toxicity (LAST), and Liposomal Bupivacaine

Michael O. On'Gele, MD, Sara Weintraub, MD, Victor Qi, MD, James Kim, MD*

KEYWORDS

- Local anesthetics • Local anesthetic toxicity • LAST • Liposomal bupivacaine
- Regional anesthesiology • Acute pain

KEY POINTS

- Local anesthetics have been transformative in the practice of anesthesiology and advancement of regional anesthesia.
- Local anesthetics are generally safe and effective; however, if a large amount of drug is injected into or absorbed into systemic circulation, this can result in toxicity.
- Local anesthetic systemic toxicity (LAST) is a rare and potentially life-threatening complication of local anesthetic administration, most notably affecting the central nervous system and cardiovascular system.
- Liposomal bupivacaine (Exparel) is perhaps the most well-known liposomal local anesthetic and uses multivesicular liposomes that ultimately result in slow degradation which has been shown to increase its duration of action up to 96 hours.
- The quest for a safe and effective ultralong-acting local anesthetic remains ongoing.

LOCAL ANESTHETICS
Background

Local anesthetics have been transformative in the practice of anesthesiology and advancement of regional anesthesia. Local anesthetics have played a vital role in the multimodal analgesia approach to patient care by decreasing the use of perioperative opioids, enhancing patient satisfaction, decreasing the incidence of postoperative nausea and vomiting, decreasing the length of hospital stay, and reducing the risk of chronic postsurgical pain.[1] The opioid-reduced anesthetic management for

Department of Anesthesiology and Critical Care, Hospital of the University of Pennsylvania, 3400 Spruce Street, Suite 680 Dulles, Philadelphia, PA 19104, USA
* Corresponding author.
E-mail address: james.kim1@pennmedicine.upenn.edu

Clin Sports Med 41 (2022) 303–315
https://doi.org/10.1016/j.csm.2021.12.001
0278-5919/22/© 2021 Elsevier Inc. All rights reserved.
sportsmed.theclinics.com

perioperative analgesia has been largely successful with the use of local anesthetics during procedures such as peripheral nerve blocks and neuraxial analgesia. Furthermore, the use of local anesthetics in the operating room and office-based procedures performed by physicians and other health care professionals rely on their predictability, safety, and efficacy. The transient blockade of motor, sensory and autonomic nerve function in neural tissue has been the hallmark of regional techniques to provide adequate depth of anesthesia or superior postoperative analgesia.[2] It has become clear that local anesthetics have many actions aside from voltage-gated sodium channel blockade. For example, they have strong anti-inflammatory effects mediated by G protein-coupled receptors which may be affected by systemic administration.[3]

Structure

The molecular structure of all local anesthetics consists of 3 components: (1) lipophilic group: aromatic benzene ring, (2) intermediate linkage: ester or amide bond, and (3) tertiary amine. Each of these structural components contributes to the biochemical properties of each local anesthetic. Local anesthetics are classified by their structure as either aminoamides or aminoesters. Aminoesters are metabolized by hydrolysis via pseudocholinesterase contained in the plasma; aminoamides undergo hepatic biotransformation via aromatic hydroxylation, N-dealkylation, and amide hydrolysis.[4] The intermediate chain of each molecule serves to classify the various local anesthetics as either esters or amides. Amide local anesthetics include bupivacaine, lidocaine, ropivacaine, mepivacaine, prilocaine, and etidocaine. Ester local anesthetics include 2-chloroprocaine, cocaine, tetracaine, and procaine. One way to readily identify to which class a local anesthetic belongs is based on the nomenclature for which the amides contain 2 "l's" in the name and esters only contain one "l." Ex. Prilocaine (Amide) versus Cocaine (Ester).

Mechanism of Action

Nerve cells are comprised of neurons with a cell membrane which creates a barrier between the Na + -rich extracellular fluid and the K + -rich intracellular fluid, creating a resting membrane potential of −60 mV to −90 mV.[5] Local anesthetics exert their effect primarily by blocking the Na + ion transit through transmembrane voltage-gated sodium channels. This ultimately results in preventing the generation of action potentials at nerve endings, blocking action potential conduction along axons in peripheral nerves, and inhibiting the depolarization-dependent release of transmitters and neuropeptides at presynaptic terminals.[6] It is important to note that local anesthetics do not alter the resting membrane potential or the threshold level of sodium channels.

It is the tertiary, lipid-soluble form of the local anesthetics which bind to the target location, the alpha subunit of the Na + channel, to exert their effect. Once the ionized form of the local anesthetic engages with the Na + channel, it is this specific binding of the alpha subunit which inactivates the Na + channel.[7] The onset of action of local anesthetics is directly related to the proportion of molecules that convert to the tertiary, lipid-soluble structure when exposed to physiologic pH (7.4).[7]

Local anesthetics have greater affinity for sodium channel receptors during their activated and inactivated states than when they are in their resting states.[8,9] There is a temporal gradation of differential blockade for which the sympathetic and sensory nerves are blocked first, followed by the smaller, unmyelinated fibers, and lastly, the larger, unmyelinated motor fibers.[10] In addition, smaller nerve fibers are generally more susceptible to blockade because a given volume of local anesthetic solution can more readily block the requisite number of sodium channels for impulse transmission to be entirely interrupted.[8,9]

Onset of Action

The onset of local anesthetics is associated with the pKa of the various local anesthetics and lipid solubility.[4] In the context of local anesthetics, the pKa can be thought of as the pH at which 50% of the molecules exist in the lipid-soluble tertiary form and 50% in the quaternary, water-soluble form.[7] Aside from benzocaine, the pKa of all other local anesthetics is > 7.4, so a greater proportion of the molecules exists in the quaternary, water-soluble form when injected into tissue with normal pH of 7.4.[7] The higher pKa's result in local anesthetic binding in their uncharged base form after injection. The closer the pKa of the local anesthetic is with respect to its surrounding pH, the faster its onset of action. An exception to this rule is 2-chloroprocaine which has the highest pKa (9.1), but has one of the quickest onset of action due to higher concentrations used (3%) without the additional risk of systemic toxicity as it is rapidly metabolized by plasma pseudocholinesterase. The onset of action for local anesthetics is also dependent on the anesthetic technique used. The shortest onset time is encountered after intrathecal or subcutaneous administration, while the longest occurs with peripheral nerve blocks.[4] In an environment with a lower pH (infected limb or abscess), the time of onset will be slower because the quaternary, water-soluble form of local anesthetic will be favored, prohibiting the local anesthetic from traveling intracellularly to bind to the sodium channels. Inflammation may disrupt local anesthetic efficacy, resulting in block failure due to increased tissue blood flow, acidic environment, and increased excitability of nerves in inflamed tissue.[3]

Potency

Local anesthetics vary in their potency, allowing for concentrations that range typically from 0.5% to 4%. This is largely due to differences in lipid solubility, which enhances diffusion through nerve sheaths and neural membranes.[7] The potency of local anesthetics correlates with lipid solubility and molecular size.

Duration of Action

The duration of action of local anesthetics is predominantly determined by their degree of protein binding. Local anesthetics reversibly bind to plasma proteins such as alpha-1-acid glycoprotein and albumin while in the plasma. In addition to protein binding, increased hydrophilicity results in faster disassociation from the lipid bilayer in an aqueous hydrophilic environment, resulting in a shorter duration of action.

Absorption

Absorption of local anesthetics is defined as the process by which the molecules move from the site of administration (intercostal, subcutaneous tissue, epidural space) into the plasma.[7] Vasopressors are added to decrease the rate of absorption and lengthen neuronal blockade. The intrinsic vasodilatory properties of certain local anesthetics affect the potency and duration of the various molecules. Vasodilation caused by local anesthetics may decrease their duration of action, but adding adjuncts such as epinephrine cause local vasoconstriction which decreases absorption and prolongs the duration of action.[7]

Distribution

Local anesthetic redistribution from blood to a variety of tissues relies on several factors: Tissue mass, perfusion, and tissue/blood partition coefficient. Immediately following the injection of local anesthetic, molecules are redistributed from the blood to highly perfused organs, such as the kidneys, lungs, brain, and heart. It is well known that local anesthetics with higher lipid solubility are associated with more tissue uptake and plasma protein binding.

Metabolism and Elimination

The elimination of local anesthetics is highly dependent on the chemical structure. Ester and amide local anesthetics differ in their mechanisms of biotransformation and excretion. The intermediate chain or linkage determines the mechanism of elimination. Esters are hydrolyzed primarily by pseudocholinesterase (butyl cholinesterase/plasma cholinesterase) yielding water-soluble metabolites that are excreted in the urine. Amide anesthetics are metabolized in the liver by hydroxylation and N-dealkylation via P-450 enzymes. The rate at which amide local anesthetics are metabolized depends on the specific local anesthetic used, but ester local anesthetics are ultimately metabolized at a faster rate.

Special Considerations of Local Anesthetics

Lidocaine, bupivacaine, and ropivacaine are some of the most commonly used local anesthetics in the perioperative setting. Various local anesthetics differ in potency and several pharmacokinetic parameters that account for differences in their onset and duration of anesthesia.[11–13] When selecting a particular local anesthetic and its concentration, several factors must be taken into consideration, including the type of procedure performed, goal for neuronal blockade (post-op analgesia vs primary anesthetic), and length of procedure.

Allergic reactions caused by local anesthetics are very rare. Immunogenic drugs are typically large in molecular weight and possess multiple valences that are recognized by immune cells.[14] Allergic reactions following local anesthetic injections are attributed to preservatives (methylparaben) or antioxidants (sulfites) contained in the solution.[15] Despite reports of cardiovascular symptoms associated with local anesthetics, like palpitations, true allergies confirmed by standardized testing are exceedingly rare, less than 1%.[16–18] Methylparaben, a preservative predominantly found in amide local anesthetics, and para-aminobenzoic acid (PABA), a preservative found in ester local anesthetics, have been shown to be the major culprits implicated in allergic reactions.[19,20] Of the 2 classes of local anesthetics, esters are more likely to result in allergic reactions, albeit extremely rare.

LOCAL ANESTHETIC SYSTEMIC TOXICITY
Introduction

Procedures involving local anesthetics are ubiquitous in medicine and are performed by a variety of medical personnel. Local anesthetics are generally safe and effective; however, if a large amount of drug is absorbed into systemic circulation from the site of therapy, supratherapeutic levels can result in toxicity. Local anesthetic systemic toxicity (LAST) is a rare and potentially life-threatening complication of local anesthetic administration, most notably affecting the central nervous system and cardiovascular system. The incidence of LAST is highly variable; recent reviews of case reports and registries have estimated its incidence as low as 0.27 per 1000 peripheral nerve blocks or as high as 1.8 per 1000 peripheral nerve blocks. Despite an increase in the number of nerve blocks performed annually, some studies have observed a downward trend in the risk of LAST.[21,22] However, this comes with the caveat that the true incidence of LAST is generally thought to be underreported. Case reports serve as a reminder that, while uncommon, practitioners should remain vigilant of the possibility of LAST and its potentially devastating consequences occurring in any patient who has received local anesthetics.

Risk Factors

The risk of developing LAST depends on patient factors, drug factors, and the site of LA administration. Most patients tolerate total body weight dosing of local anesthetics; however, patients at the extremes of age are at increased risk of LAST.[21] Skeletal muscle represents a significant volume of distribution for systemically absorbed local anesthetic, therefore neonates, infants, and the elderly can be at increased risk due to comparatively low lean body mass. Neonates and infants also have lower levels of plasma proteins which bind local anesthetics, allowing for a higher concentration of unbound drug which exerts a clinical effect. Whereas the elderly may be at increased risk due to comorbidities (particularly renal, hepatic, and cardiac disease) which may affect drug metabolism/clearance and render them more susceptible to the toxic effects of local anesthetics.

Different local anesthetics have varying levels of potency which influences their levels of toxicity. This results in not only different maximum dosages, but also variable presentation, with some more likely to present with cardiovascular symptoms and others with neurologic symptoms. The cardiovascular collapse/CNS dose ratio can be used to compare the relative cardiovascular or neurologic toxicity of local anesthetics. For example, bupivacaine is one of the most potent local anesthetics and the most difficult to treat when LAST occurs.[21] Bupivacaine is more likely to present with cardiovascular toxicity compared with the less potent lidocaine which is more likely to present with neurologic toxicity.[23] Local anesthetics also have variable intrinsic dose-dependent vasoactivity which affects the rate of systemic absorption. Although they generally act as vasodilators, ropivacaine and mepivacaine have mild vasoconstriction properties at low doses which may reduce systemic absorption, whereas lidocaine and bupivacaine act entirely as vasodilators which may increase the rate of systemic absorption.[24,25] Liposomal local anesthetics such as liposomal bupivacaine (Exparel) are formulated to allow for slow release of the local anesthetic and delayed absorption into systemic circulation. A literature search of PubMed did not yield any case reports of LAST in the setting of liposomal bupivacaine administration and a prior retrospective review of randomized controlled trials involving liposomal bupivacaine did not identify any definitive instances of LAST.[26] However, analysis of data from the FDA Adverse Event Reporting System which does not have a code specific to LAST has identified a pharmacovigilance signal indicating an association between LAST and Exparel.[27] Regardless of the selected local anesthetic, higher doses are associated with a higher risk of LAST.[28] Furthermore, the toxicity of local anesthetics is additive and thus continuous catheter-based techniques are associated with a higher risk of LAST. The site of injection and the vascularity of the site also modify the risk; high vascularity may allow for increased systemic absorption of local anesthetic. Direct intravascular injection of local anesthetic results in the highest systemic uptake and therefore, the highest risk of LAST. Paravertebral and intercostal nerve blocks were classically reported to have the next highest risk of systemic absorption followed in descending order by epidural, brachial plexus blocks, and subcutaneous injection. However, more recent studies have observed LAST occurring 4 to 5 times more often with peripheral nerve blocks compared with epidural, with the highest incidence observed with paravertebral blocks followed by upper extremity blocks and none after lower extremity blocks.[23,28] LAST has also been observed in the setting of newer techniques such as fascial plane blocks (ie, transversus abdominis plane (TAP), pectoral, or quadratus lumborum blocks) and local infiltration analgesia in total joint arthroplasty, both of which are high volume techniques.[29] A study of peak local anesthetic serum concentration following local infiltration analgesia indicates that absorption is higher in total hip arthroplasty than total knee arthroplasty and on average results in higher absorption when compared with the femoral nerve block.[30]

Presentation

LAST is a clinical diagnosis and seizure is the most common symptom (60%–70% according to some studies).[21] The classic presentation of LAST begins with prodromal symptoms such as lightheadedness, dizziness, tinnitus, visual disturbances, and perioral numbness within a few minutes after an injection of local anesthetic. The onset of symptoms within 1 minute is suggestive of intravascular injection while onset within 5 minutes is suggestive of partial intravascular injection or tissue absorption. These symptoms can quickly progress to seizure or loss of consciousness, followed by arrhythmias, hypotension, or cardiac arrest. However, recent analyses have observed that approximately one-third of reported cases present atypically. These cases either presented with isolated cardiovascular symptoms or occurred at least 5 minutes after administration.[23] Other atypical presentations include the simultaneous onset of cardiovascular and neurologic symptoms. The most recent American Society of Regional Anesthesia and Pain Medicine (ASRA) practice advisory on LAST has observed a continued shift of LAST toward delayed presentation with a significant number of cases presenting between 11 and 60 minutes after injection and in some cases, over an hour.[30] The symptoms of LAST may closely resemble other perioperative complications or be obscured by sedation, so care must be taken to ensure timely diagnosis.

Prevention

Prevention of LAST is a multifactorial process; no single intervention has been demonstrated to eliminate the risk. Ultrasound guidance greatly reduces the incidence of LAST following a peripheral nerve block with one study observing a 65% reduction; however, the risk is not eliminated and LAST has been described in the setting of ultrasound use.[28] Incremental injection and intermittent aspiration can also reduce the risk of LAST by detecting unintentional needle tip migration and increasing the amount of time over which the local anesthetic is injected. Dose fractionation by incremental injection reduces the maximum serum concentration and allows for the proceduralist to abort without giving the entire planned dose if early signs of toxicity are detected.[31] However, the incidence of a false negative aspiration is estimated to be 2%.[30] The current ASRA practice guideline also recommends using the lowest effective dose of local anesthetic and using an intravascular marker such as epinephrine if a potentially toxic dose is planned.[30] Although local anesthetics are commonly dosed by total body weight, current guidelines also recommend special considerations for truncal fascial plane blocks including using lower concentrations, dosing on lean body weight, and using epinephrine to reduce the risk of LAST.[30]

Management

Practice guidelines on the management of LAST are maintained and periodically updated by ASRA. If LAST is suspected, any further administration of local anesthetic should immediately be stopped and help should be obtained. The successful treatment of LAST is highly dependent on airway management and adequate oxygenation and ventilation because hypoxia, hypercapnia, and acidosis can exacerbate LAST and interfere with resuscitation.[30] This potentiation of LAST may be due to increased ion trapping of local anesthetic within myocytes and neurons, increased free fraction of local anesthetic, or worsening myocardial depression. The current ASRA guideline recommends early administration of intravenous lipid emulsion to manage severe LAST which may manifest with arrhythmias, prolonged seizures, or rapid clinical deterioration.[30] The use of lipid emulsion for the treatment of LAST is an off-label indication and tends to be well tolerated.[30] Intravenous lipid helps resuscitate patients by scavenging and accelerating redistribution of local anesthetic in addition to increasing cardiac output via vasoconstriction and direct cardiotonic effects; these mechanisms are most effective when lipid is administered early and the local anesthetic is at peak plasma concentration.[32] Before the introduction of lipid therapy, management of last was limited to seizure management, advanced cardiac life support (ACLS), and cardiopulmonary bypass.

Lipid emulsion therapy uses 20% intravenous lipid emulsion and has been simplified to total body weight dosing.[33] The timeliness of administration is the most important and the order of administration is not critical. Patients weighing more than 70 kg should receive a bolus of 100 mL over 2 to 3 minutes and an infusion of ~250 mg over 15 to 20 minutes. Patients weighing less than 70 kg should receive a bolus of 1.5 mL/kg over 2 to 3 minutes and an infusion of 0.25 mL/kg/min. If the patient remains unstable after these interventions, the bolus dose should be repeated and the infusion rate doubled. Propofol is not an appropriate agent for lipid therapy due to a comparatively low concentration of lipids and its myocardial depressant activity.

Seizures may exacerbate metabolic derangements and timely management is crucial. Benzodiazepines are first-line therapy for seizures due to their relatively stable hemodynamic profile. Propofol may be used if other agents are unavailable or contraindicated but, should be conducted with low doses and extreme caution due to its hemodynamic effects. If seizures are refractory to therapy, neuromuscular blockade can be considered to minimize metabolic derangements.[30]

Patients who suffer cardiac arrest in the setting of LAST should also promptly receive ACLS. However, it is important to note that the standard ACLS dose of epinephrine can impair resuscitation in the setting of LAST; therefore initially small doses of ≤ 1 μg/kg are preferred.[30] Amiodarone is highly preferred if ventricular arrhythmias develop, and lidocaine should be avoided. Vasopressin, calcium channel blockers, and beta-blockers are also not recommended. Lastly, cardiopulmonary bypass should be considered if the patient fails to respond to lipid and vasopressor therapy.

As with all medical emergencies, it is important to obtain and maintain intravenous access. If intravenous access cannot be obtained, intraosseous access is acceptable. Once stability has been achieved, an infusion of intravenous lipid emulsion should be continued for at least another 15 minutes. Afterward, patients should be observed for a minimum of 2 hours if only isolated neurologic symptoms occurred or 4 to 6 hours if cardiovascular instability occurred. LAST is a potentially life-threatening event and it is important that practitioners who use local anesthetics are aware of the risk factors, presentation, and management.

LIPOSOMAL BUPIVACAINE
Introduction

Local anesthetics (LA) are relatively small-sized molecules that can be easily absorbed into the bloodstream and removed from their desired sites of action. In the setting of peripheral nerve blocks, even the intermediate-acting LA bupivacaine and ropivacaine have been shown to only provide patients about 8 to 12 hours of analgesia, resulting in increased pain the night of their surgery once the nerve block wears off.[34] The ability to prolong the duration of action of local anesthetics has thus been a topic of great interest in the field of regional anesthesia.

The earliest efforts to accomplish this goal included the use of additives to LA formulations and the use of continuous peripheral nerve catheters. Epinephrine is the most commonly used adjunct for short and intermediate-acting LAs, with some studies demonstrating a 200% increase in the duration of action (for lidocaine, this would prolong a 1–2 hour block to approximately 3–6 hours).[35] Unfortunately, there has been limited evidence demonstrating such an effect with longer-acting LA.[36] Additionally, there have been concerns regarding neurotoxicity due to epinephrine's direct effect on alpha-1-adrenergic receptors, resulting in cerebral vasoconstriction. This particular concern is especially heightened in patients with a history of smoking, hypertension, and diabetes mellitus who are already at a higher risk for neural toxicity.[37] Buprenorphine and dexamethasone have been 2 of the most effective additives to long-acting LAs studied thus far, but even their ability to prolong the duration of action is modest at best, increasing the duration to 18 and 22 hours for interscalene brachial plexus blocks, when combined with bupivacaine or ropivacaine, respectively.[38,39]

Continuous peripheral nerve catheters may certainly extend the duration of analgesia, but they also present many disadvantages. Compared with single-shot injections, they are more costly, susceptible to pump malfunctions, may require additional expertise in placement and maintenance, and are associated with high rates of catheter migration.[34] In fact, one study of 20 volunteers receiving either interscalene or femoral nerve catheters demonstrated catheter dislodgment rates of 5% and 25%, respectively, within 6 hours following regular physical exercises.[40] Additionally, while an extremely rare occurrence, infection leading to sepsis and even death remains a concern.[34]

Background

The search for a safe, long-acting local anesthetic has led to the development of liposomal formulations. Liposomes are microscopic structures that consist of an aqueous core surrounded by at least one phospholipid bilayer. Liposomal Bupivacaine (Exparel), created by Pacira Pharmaceuticals, is perhaps the most well-known liposomal local anesthetic and uses multivesicular liposomes (DepoFoam delivery system) containing bupivacaine. DepoFoam has a non-concentric shape that ultimately results in slow degradation through internal fusion and division.[41] This slow degradation process has been shown to increase its duration of action to 96 hours and 120 hours for local infiltration and interscalene nerve blocks, respectively.

Liposomal bupivacaine was first approved by the FDA in 2011 for surgical field infiltration only after 2 studies demonstrated efficacy in hemorrhoidectomy and bunionectomy surgeries compared with placebo. It was not until 2018 that Exparel gained approval for use in interscalene brachial plexus blocks. As of now, the interscalene block is still the only peripheral nerve block for which Exparel is approved for "on-label" use. Intended as a single shot injection, it is recommended that no greater than 20 mL (266 mg) and 10 mL (133 mg) be used for local surgical field infiltration and interscalene blocks, respectively. Nausea, vomiting, constipation, and pyrexia are the most common side effects, with greater than 10% incidence. The manufacturers of Exparel warn against mixing their formulation with nonbupivacaine LAs such as lidocaine as this can result in immediate release of bupivacaine molecules with the potential for life-threatening cardiovascular and central nervous system toxicity. It is recommended that injection of Exparel should be delayed at least 20-min following lidocaine injection and that no additional local anesthetics should be given within

96 hours. Exparel should not be mixed with hypotonic solutions or water, as this may also disrupt the liposomal structure, and it should not make contact with any antiseptics, such as betadine. Exparel may be mixed with nonliposomal bupivacaine in a ratio not exceeding 2:1 and may be diluted with normotonic solutions such as normal saline or lactated ringers in a maximum ratio of 1:14 (0.89 mg/mL), usually with the purpose of injecting a greater overall volume.

Exparel's indication for interscalene nerve blocks comes from one study involving 155 patients undergoing total shoulder arthroplasty or rotator cuff surgery, which demonstrated improvement in pain scores, opioid consumption, median time to opioid rescue, and percentage of opioid-free patients compared with placebo.[42] It is important to note that the investigators of this study did not compare Exparel to plain bupivacaine. The only specific contraindication mentioned on the Exparel package insert regards the use of liposomal bupivacaine in obstetric paracervical nerve blocks, which has been shown to result in fetal bradycardia and death.[43] Due to the current lack of pertinent studies regarding safety and efficacy, Exparel is not recommended for epidural, intrathecal, intravascular, and intraarticular injections nor in pregnant or pediatric patients.

Current Evidence

While numerous studies have demonstrated Exparel's efficacy compared with placebo in reducing pain and opioid consumption, these studies that led to its FDA approval did not compare its use to plain bupivacaine. Two recently published systematic reviews from February 2021 focused specifically on this topic. A meta-analysis by Hussain and colleagues compared the efficacy of perineural Exparel to plain bupivacaine or ropivacaine with respect to analgesic outcomes, postsurgical pain, quality of life, and opioid dependence.[43] Nine RCTs involving 619 patients ultimately met the authors' inclusion criteria. The included studies involved patients receiving intercostal, pectoral myofascial plane, fascia iliaca, dorsal penile, interscalene, or adductor canal nerve blocks. Perineural Exparel resulted in a statistically significant reduction in rest pain over 24 through 72 hours versus plain bupivacaine and ropivacaine (the primary outcome); however, the difference in pain scores failed to meet the authors' threshold for clinical significance.[43] Additionally, when the authors excluded one industry-sponsored RCT from their analysis, this difference became statistically insignificant. There were no differences in opioid consumption over 72-h, time to first analgesic request, opioid-related side effects, length of hospital stay, functional recovery, or persistent pain at 30 days between patients receiving liposomal versus plain bupivacaine.[43] Patient satisfaction was found to be higher in the liposomal bupivacaine group.[43] The authors offered one plausible explanation as to why liposomal bupivacaine demonstrated no additional benefits compared with the non-liposomal formulation: Immediately following bupivacaine injection, local tissue inflammation occurs, resulting in an acidotic medium that prevents further liposomal bupivacaine from penetrating the cellular bilayer and acting on the intracellular voltage-gated sodium channel.[43]

A second systematic review by Jin and colleagues yielded similarly negative results. Their study included 13 RCTs comparing the use of liposomal bupivacaine to traditional perineural local anesthetics with respect to opioid use and pain scores. Patients received TAP blocks in 6 of these RCTs, adductor canal blocks in 2 RCTs, brachial plexus blocks in 3 RCTs, fascia iliaca block in 1 RCT, and ankle block in 1 RCT.[44] Although 4 of the 6 RCTs involving TAP blocks reported a longer duration of action with Exparel, the authors were concerned about reliability of these studies given generally small sample sizes, conflicts of interest, and high risk of bias scores.[44] There were conflicting results from the 3 RCTs involving brachial plexus blocks, and all but one of the other RCTs involving alternate types of perineural blocks reported negative findings.[44] Jin and colleagues concluded that "there is currently little evidence that in regional anesthesia, liposomal bupivacaine significantly prolongs the duration of analgesia compared to conventional local anesthetics."[44] The authors also offered a hypothesis as to why surgical site infiltration with Exparel compared with plain bupivacaine has been shown to be effective whereas regional anesthesia with Exparel has not: Nerves targeted in regional block techniques are larger than those targeted with local infiltration. There must be a high enough concentration and gradient of free bupivacaine surrounding the nerve in order for the local anesthetics to diffuse through the epineurium and perineurium. The authors suggested that after its initial injection and due to the slow-release technology, liposomal bupivacaine may not release enough free bupivacaine molecules at the same time to create a high enough concentration gradient.[44] The authors also noted that factors such as surgical procedure, site of block, and tissue vascularity may influence efficacy as some studies have demonstrated no additional benefit of locally infiltrated Exparel in total knee replacement surgery, laparoscopic urologic surgery, and breast surgery.[44–47]

Although Exparel is the most commonly used and perhaps only clinically relevant long-acting formulation of bupivacaine, others are under development. HTX-011 is a new drug being developed by Heron Therapeutics and consists of slow-release bupivacaine as well as meloxicam, encapsulated in a bioerodable polymer (Biochronomer) which releases these drugs over 72 hours.[41] The company is also producing a mepivacaine-containing formulation called APF112 using this Biochronomer technology.[41] HTX-011 has undergone two phase III trials. The first study compared its efficacy to plain bupivacaine and to placebo for local infiltration during bunionectomy surgery, while the second included patients undergoing open inguinal herniorrhaphy with mesh. HTX-011 showed a statistically significant reduction in opioid consumption as well as pain intensity scores in both trials.[48,49] Despite these findings, neither HTX-011 nor APF112 is yet FDA-approved.

DURECT Corporation and Sandoz AG are currently developing POSIMIR, which is an extended-release formulation of bupivacaine using SABER-bupivacaine (sucrose acetate isobutyrate extended-release) technology. Sucrose acetate isobutyrate (SAIB) is a biodegradable depot that allows for high concentration bupivacaine storage. Because the drug contains benzyl alcohol, it is not designed for perineural use due to concern for neurotoxicity. After infiltration into the target tissue, POSIMIR releases bupivacaine at a rate of about 10 mg/h over 72 hours. POSIMIR's phase III trial consisted of patients undergoing laparoscopic cholecystectomy and open laparotomy. POSIMIR demonstrated a significant reduction in pain intensity on movement scores but not in overall opioid consumption compared with bupivacaine.[50]

SUMMARY

The quest for a safe and effective ultralong-acting local anesthetic remains ongoing. The excitement that came after Exparel's FDA approval may have been tempered by the recent systematic reviews questioning its advantages over traditional local anesthetics in regional anesthesia. Still, liposomal bupivacaine may be a more favorable option for surgical field blocks, and indeed, it remains as a component in intraoperative protocols for hip fracture surgery at many institutions despite this limited evidence.

DISCLOSURE

The authors have nothing to disclose.

REFERENCES

1. David MD, Jeffrey LA. Local Anesthetic Systemic Toxicity. Aesthet Surg J 2014; 34(7):1111–9.
2. Morgan GE, Mikhail MS, Murray MJ. Clinical anesthesiology. New York: Lange Medical Books/McGraw Hill Medical Pub. Division.; 2006. p. 261–74.
3. Lirk P, Hollmann MW, Strichartz G. The science of local anesthesia: basic research, clinical application, and future directions. Anesth Analg 2018;126(4): 1381–92.
4. Heavner JE. Local anesthetics. Curr Opin Anaesthesiol 2007;20:336–42.
5. Faust's Anesthesiology Review. In: Trentman TL, Gaitan BD, Gali B, et al, editors. Faust's anesthesiology review. 5th edition; 2020. p. 279–80.
6. Brull SJ, Greene NM. Time-courses of zones of differential sensory blockade during spinal anesthesia with hyperbaric tetracaine or bupivacaine. Anesth Analg 1989;69:342–7.
7. Becker DE, Kenneth LR. Local anesthetics: review of pharmacological considerations. Anesth Prog 2012;59(2):90–101 [quiz: 102-3].
8. Berde CB, Strichartz GR. Local anesthetics. In: Miller RD, Eriksson LI, Fleisher LA, et al, editors. Miller's anesthesia. 7th edition. Philadelphia (PA): Elsevier, Churchill Livingstone; 2009.
9. Katzung BG, White PF. Local anesthetics. In: Katzung BG, Masters SB, Trevor AJ, editors. Basic and clinical pharmacology. 11th edition. New York: McGraw-Hill Companies Inc; 2009. 2–2.
10. Jaffe RA, Rowe MA. Differential nerve block. Direct measurement on individual myelinated and unmyelinated dorsal root axons. Anesthesiology 1996;84(6): 1455–64.
11. Morris R, McKay W, Mushlin P. Comparison of pain associated with intradermal and subcutaneous infiltration with various local anesthetic solutions. Anesth Analg 1987;66(11):1180–2.
12. Wahl MJ, Overton D, Howell J, et al. Pain on injection of prilocaine plain vs. lidocaine with epinephrine. A prospective double-blind study. J Am Dent Assoc 2001;132:1396–401.
13. Wahl MJ, Schmitt MM, Overton DA, et al. Injection pain of bupivacaine with epinephrine vs. prilocaine plain. J Am Dent Assoc 2002;133:1652–6.
14. Adkinson NF Jr. Drug allergy. In: Adkinson NF Jr, Yunginger JW, Busse WW, et al, editors. Middleton's allergy: principles and practice. 6th edition. Philadelphia (PA): Mosby Inc; 2003.
15. Schatz M. Adverse reactions to local anesthetics. Immunol Allergy Clin N Am 1992;12:585–609.
16. Ring J, Franz R, Brockow K. Anaphylactic reactions to local anesthetics. Chem Immunol Allergy 2010;95:190–200.
17. Berkun Y, Ben-Zvi A, Levy Y, et al. Evaluation of adverse reactions to local anesthetics: experience with 236 patients. Ann Allergy Asthma Immunol 2003;91: 342–5.
18. Batinac T, Sotošek Tokmadžić V, Peharda V, et al. Adverse reactions and alleged allergy to local anesthetics: analysis of 331 patients. J Dermatol 2013;40:522–7.
19. Eggleston ST, Lush LW. Understanding allergic reactions to local anesthetics. Ann Pharmacother 1996;30:851–7.
20. Brull R, McCartney CJ, Chan VW, et al. Neurological complications after regional anesthesia: contemporary estimates of risk. Anesth Analg 2007;104:965–74.

21. Gitman M, Barrington MJ. Local anesthetic systemic toxicity: a review of recent case reports and registries. Reg Anesth Pain Med 2018;43(2):124–30.
22. Mörwald EE, Zubizarreta N, Cozowicz C, et al. Incidence of local anesthetic systemic toxicity in orthopedic patients receiving peripheral nerve blocks. Reg Anesth Pain Med 2017;42(4):442–5.
23. Neal JM, Bernards CM, Butterworth JF, et al. ASRA practice advisory on local anesthetic systemic toxicity. Reg Anesth Pain Med 2010;35(2):152–61.
24. Guinard JP, Carpenter RL, Morell RC. Effect of local anesthetic concentration on capillary blood flow in human skin. Reg Anesth J Neural Blockade Obstet Surg Pain Control 1992;17(6):317–21.
25. Ishiyama T, Dohi S, Iida H, et al. The effects of topical and intravenous ropivacaine on canine pial microcirculation. Anesth Analg 1997;85(1):75–81.
26. Ilfeld BM, Viscusi ER, Hadzic A, et al. Safety and side effect profile of liposome bupivacaine (Exparel) in peripheral nerve blocks. Reg Anesth Pain Med 2015;40(5):572–82.
27. Aggarwal N. Local anesthetics systemic toxicity association with exparel (bupivacaine liposome)-a pharmacovigilance evaluation. Expert Opin Drug Saf 2018;17(6):581–7.
28. Barrington MJ, Kluger R. Ultrasound guidance reduces the risk of local anesthetic systemic toxicity following peripheral nerve blockade. Reg Anesth Pain Med 2013;38(4):289–99.
29. Affas F. Local infiltration analgesia in knee and hip arthroplasty efficacy and safety. Scand J pain 2016;13:59–66.
30. Neal JM, Barrington MJ, Fettiplace MR, et al. The third American Society of regional anesthesia and pain medicine practice advisory on local anesthetic systemic toxicity: executive summary 2017. Reg Anesth Pain Med 2018;43(2):113–23.
31. Mather LE, Copeland SE, Ladd LA. Acute toxicity of local anesthetics: underlying pharmacokinetic and pharmacodynamic concepts. Reg Anesth Pain Med 2005;30(6):553–66.
32. Fettiplace MR, Weinberg G. The mechanisms underlying lipid resuscitation therapy. Reg Anesth Pain Med 2018;43(2):138–49.
33. Neal JM, Neal EJ, Weinberg GL. American Society of regional anesthesia and pain medicine local anesthetic systemic toxicity checklist: 2020 version. Reg Anesth Pain Med 2021;46(1):81–2.
34. Chahar P, Cummings KC III. Liposomal bupivacaine: A review of a new bupivacaine formulation. J pain Res 2012;5:257.
35. Liu S, Carpenter RL, Chiu AA, et al. Epinephrine prolongs duration of subcutaneous infiltration of local anesthesia in a dose-related manner:: Correlation with magnitude of vasoconstriction. Reg Anesth J Neural Blockade Obstet Surg Pain Control 1995;20(5):378–84.
36. Weber A, Fournier R, Van Gessel E, et al. Epinephrine does not prolong the analgesia of 20 mL ropivacaine 0.5% or 0.2% in a femoral three-in-one block. Anesth Analg 2001;93(5):1327–31.
37. Brummett CM, Williams BA. Additives to local anesthetics for peripheral nerve blockade. Int Anesthesiol Clin 2011;49(4):104.
38. Cummings KC III, Napierkowski DE, Parra-Sanchez I, et al. Effect of dexamethasone on the duration of interscalene nerve blocks with ropivacaine or bupivacaine. Br J Anaesth 2011;107(3):446–53.
39. Kosel J, Bobik P, Tomczyk M. Buprenorphine–the unique opioid adjuvant in regional anesthesia. Expert Rev Clin Pharmacol 2016;9(3):375–83.

40. Marhofer D, Marhofer P, Triffterer L, et al. Dislocation rates of perineural catheters: A volunteer study. Br J Anaesth 2013;111(5):800–6.
41. Coppens SJR, Zawodny Z, Dewinter G, et al. In search of the holy grail: Poisons and extended release local anesthetics. Best Pract Res Clin Anaesthesiology 2019;33(1):3–21. Available at: https://www-sciencedirect-com.proxy.library.upenn.edu/science/article/pii/S1521689619300072.
42. Patel MA, Gadsden JC, Nedeljkovic SS, et al. Brachial plexus block with liposomal bupivacaine for shoulder surgery improves analgesia and reduces opioid consumption: Results from a multicenter, randomized, double-blind, controlled trial. Pain Med 2020;21(2):387–400.
43. Hussain N, Brull R, Sheehy B, et al. Perineural liposomal bupivacaine is not superior to nonliposomal bupivacaine for peripheral nerve block AnalgesiaA systematic review and meta-analysis. Anesthesiology 2021;134(2):147–64.
44. Jin Z, Ding O, Islam A, et al. Comparison of liposomal bupivacaine and conventional local anesthetic agents in regional anesthesia: a systematic review. Anesth Analg 2021;132(6):1626–34.
45. Tan P, Martin M, Shank N, et al. A comparison of four analgesic regimens for acute postoperative pain control in breast augmentation patients. Ann Plast Surg 2017;78(6):S299.
46. Knight RB, Walker PW, Keegan KA, et al. A randomized controlled trial for pain control in laparoscopic urologic surgery: 0.25% bupivacaine versus long-acting liposomal bupivacaine. J endourology 2015;29(9):1019–24.
47. Schroer WC, Diesfeld PG, LeMarr AR, et al. Does extended-release liposomal bupivacaine better control pain than bupivacaine after total knee arthroplasty (TKA)? A prospective, randomized clinical trial. J Arthroplasty 2015;30(9):64–7.
48. Viscusi E, Gimbel JS, Pollack RA, et al. HTX-011 reduced pain intensity and opioid consumption versus bupivacaine HCl in bunionectomy: Phase III results from the randomized epoch 1 study. Reg Anesth Pain Med 2019;44(7):700–6.
49. Viscusi E, Minkowitz H, Winkle P, et al. HTX-011 reduced pain intensity and opioid consumption versus bupivacaine HCl in herniorrhaphy: results from the phase 3 epoch 2 study. Hernia 2019;23(6):1071–80.
50. Gan TJ, Papaconstantinou H, Durieux M, et al. Treatment of postoperative pain in major abdominal surgery with SABER®-bupivacaine: Results of the BESST trial. Pain 2014;6(7):8–9.

Continuous Catheter Techniques

Brittany Deiling, DO*, Kenneth Mullen, MD, Ashley M. Shilling, MD

KEYWORDS

- Nerve block • Peripheral catheter • Regional anesthesia • Ambulatory surgery
- Infusion pump

KEY POINTS

- For painful orthopedic surgery, continuous peripheral nerve catheters are indicated when a prolonged neural block is desired beyond the duration of a single-shot nerve block injection.
- Continuous catheters have been shown to promote better postoperative analgesia, increase patient satisfaction, and have a positive influence on both surgical outcomes and rehabilitation compared with other modalities.
- Peripheral nerve catheters provide flexibility in terms of both duration of nerve block and density by controlling the dose and concentration of the local anesthetic infusate.
- The key to safe at-home nerve catheters is proper patient selection, willingness of the patient to accept responsibility for the catheter, and appropriate patient education and resources.

INTRODUCTION

Continuous peripheral nerve block (CPNB) catheters are simple in concept: percutaneously inserting a catheter adjacent to a peripheral nerve. This procedure is followed by local anesthetic infusion via the catheter that can be titrated to effect for extended anesthesia or analgesia in the perioperative period. The reported benefits of peripheral nerve catheters used in the surgical population include improved pain scores, decreased narcotic use, decreased nausea/vomiting, decreased pruritus, decreased sedation, improved sleep, and improved patient satisfaction. The first report of peripheral nerve catheter use in the United States was in 1946 and was placed to prolong upper extremity surgical anesthesia using a needle through a cork taped to the patient's chest.[1] CPNBs have evolved over decades from experimental case reports to validated studies that are widely accepted by the medical community. Reports show uses for treatment of intractable hiccups,[2] for treatment of vasospasm due to

Department of Anesthesiology, University of Virginia Health System, PO Box 800710, Charlottesville, VA 22908-0710, USA
* Corresponding author.
E-mail address: bd8hp@hscmail.mcc.virginia.edu

Clin Sports Med 41 (2022) 317–328
https://doi.org/10.1016/j.csm.2021.11.011
0278-5919/22/Published by Elsevier Inc.
sportsmed.theclinics.com

Raynaud disease,[3] to induce sympathectomy and produce vasodilation for traumatic vascular injury,[4] for digit/extremity replantation,[5] and for the treatment of peripheral embolism.[6] There are other reports of the use of peripheral nerve catheters in chronic pain conditions including chronic regional pain syndrome[7] and postamputation phantom limb pain.[8] In the setting of orthopedic trauma, peripheral nerve block catheters can be used for analgesia during patient transport to the surgical institution and during the time of awaiting surgical fixation.[9]

Nevertheless, most continuous peripheral nerve catheter use is during the perioperative setting for prolonged postoperative analgesia. Since its origin, continuous peripheral nerve catheters were used in the hospital setting with direct patient monitoring and nursing care of the catheter and infusion. In 1997, the first ambulatory peripheral nerve catheter was described using a portable home infusion pump, and since then, almost every anatomic catheter location has been reported in ambulatory settings.[9]

INDICATIONS FOR PERIPHERAL NERVE CATHETERS

The main indication for continuous peripheral nerve catheters is when a prolonged neural block is desired beyond the duration of action of a single nerve block injection. CPNBs have been suggested to be beneficial in a variety of medical implications, but the published randomized controlled trials have exclusively studied postoperative patients. The main benefit of nerve catheters is analgesia, with greatest effects in surgical sites that are completely innervated by nerves targeted by the local anesthesia infusion. These sites include the foot with a sciatic catheter and the shoulder with an interscalene brachial plexus catheter.[9] On the other hand, a single peripheral nerve catheter for surgical sites innervated by multiple nerves, such as orthopedic procedures on the hip, knee, and ankle, can expect to provide incomplete analgesia and necessitate the use of adjuvant analgesics or multiple catheters.

Patients undergoing orthopedic surgical procedures with anticipated considerable and prolonged pain should be considered for a CPNB. Other indications include surgical pain not easily treated with less invasive analgesic techniques, opioid-tolerant patients, or intolerance to oral analgesic regimens.[9] For both upper and lower extremity orthopedic surgery, continuous catheters have been shown to promote better postoperative analgesia, increase patient satisfaction, and to positively influence both surgical outcome and rehabilitation compared with intravenous opioids.[10] CPNB catheters are advantageous because of fewer side effects when compared with intravenous opioids and patient-controlled analgesia. Furthermore, CPNBs have safety benefits when compared with central neuraxial techniques for patients on anticoagulants.[11]

Orthopedic surgery is considered one of the most painful surgeries, causing significantly increased pains scores for 2 to 3 days postoperatively.[12] Furthermore, acute postsurgical pain that is intense and persistent is a risk factor for the development of chronic pain. In questionnaire-based postoperative evaluations after hip and knee arthroplasty, 28% of patients after hip arthroplasty and 33% of patients after knee arthroplasty report suffering from chronic pain.[13,14] Implementing a postsurgical analgesia plan that includes a peripheral nerve catheter for painful procedures could be an important factor for decreasing the risk of chronic pain development.[15]

BENEFITS OF CONTINUOUS CATHETERS FOR ORTHOPEDIC PATIENTS

Although the benefits of single-shot peripheral nerve blocks are well established in the postoperative period, single-shot nerve blocks typically wear off between 12 to

24 hours and the resultant escalation of pain can be significant, particularly for patients who are recovering at home without access to intravenous pain medications. The concept of rebound pain, or hyperalgesia after a nerve block has resolved, has garnered significant attention over the past years.[16] Although mechanisms are still being determined, the phenomenon may be, in part, from abnormal spontaneous C-fiber hyperactivity and nociceptor hyperexcitability following a nerve block, even in the absence of any neurologic injury.[17,18] This period of hyperalgesia can be distressing to patients and may lead to patient dissatisfaction with regional anesthesia and could even deter patients from future peripheral nerve blocks. Interestingly, unplanned physician visits in the first 48 hours following wrist surgery was greater in patients receiving brachial plexus blocks than those who received general anesthesia without a nerve block.[19] CPNB catheters serve the important purpose of extending the duration of analgesia throughout the most painful portion of the postoperative period and can delay the onset of postsurgical pain until inflammation has decreased and the healing process has progressed.

Most of the published literature on the outcomes of continuous catheter techniques focuses on analgesia benefits including reduced pain scores and decreased analgesic requirements. Almost every nerve catheter site including brachial plexus, femoral, adductor canal, and sciatic demonstrates analgesic benefit when compared with other pain modalities including patient-controlled analgesia, wound infiltration, and single-shot peripheral nerve block.[20–22] Outcomes including pain scores at various time points, first time to opioids, and total opioids have been shown to be positively impacted by CPNBs. Surgeries such as rotator cuff repair and ligament reconstruction of the knee can lead to significant pain for patients. Even for healthy sports medicine patients, pain can be disabling and create poor quality of life and sleep disturbances in the postoperative days. For this reason, CPNBs are becoming a mainstay of many orthopedic surgeries, both for inpatient and in ambulatory patients.

While analgesic benefits are the primary outcome studied in patients receiving CPNB, functional outcomes play a significant role in the postoperative period and deserve greater focus for research. Continuous femoral nerve catheters served for decades as the "go to" technique for patients undergoing total knee arthroplasty (TKA). In addition to offering significant analgesic benefits, femoral catheters offer functional benefits to patients including improved range of motion.[23] Improved joint flexion has been demonstrated in patients undergoing TKA up to 6 months postoperatively.[24,25] Literature on the adductor canal block was published in 2011 with the finding that it preserved quadriceps function while proving significant analgesic benefit.[26] Since that time, more studies support the analgesic benefit of adductor blocks with improved mobilization including standing, sitting, ambulation, and climbing stairs.[27,28] Although functional outcome studies are most commonly performed in patients undergoing TKA, one pilot study demonstrated improved shoulder range of motion up to 12 weeks in patients undergoing surgery for adhesive capsulitis.[29] Further research is needed on the long-term functional outcome benefits of CPNBs.

In addition to pain outcomes, CPNBs have also improved quality-of=life outcomes. One notable benefit includes improved sleep postoperatively in patients undergoing shoulder surgery receiving a continuous interscalene catheter.[30] Decreased opioid side effects like pruritus, nausea and vomiting, and sedation have also been demonstrated in patients receiving a continuous nerve catheter.[31–33] Patient satisfaction and quality of recovery is a critical area of focus in the postoperative period and should be noted as an important benefit of an analgesic regimen.

CPNBs allow greater flexibility for dosing and greater titration of analgesia while potentially sparing a dense motor block; this may be particularly helpful in patients at risk for compartment syndrome.[32] Furthermore, a continuous catheter can allow for intermittent neurologic examinations after a surgery, followed by a bolus or restarting of a local anesthetic infusion. Nerve catheters allow for elegant titration of local anesthetics to meet the needs of patients and can also be titrated to the outcomes of physical therapy.

Continuous catheters have allowed what once were inpatient surgeries to be performed in an ambulatory setting. Total joint arthroplasty surgeries, including total knee, hip, and shoulder, are now commonly performed in ambulatory surgical centers with patients being discharged home comfortably with continuous catheters. Patients undergoing foot and ankle surgery as well as upper extremity surgery are ideal for same-day discharge with continuous catheters for analgesic management. With patient and family education, patients can be easily taught to manage their infusions including patient-controlled bolus options. Catheter removal is simple, and many disposable pump options allow patients to simply discard their devices after use.

In addition to the benefits noted earlier, cost savings cannot be overlooked because financial outcomes are imperative to providing cost-effective quality care. CPNBs have been shown to reduce time until patient discharge readiness as well as shorten recovery length of stay.[9,34] Studies randomizing patients receiving CPNB to home or hospital recovery have shown no difference in outcomes other than cost savings in the home-CPNB patients.[35,36] In addition to those noted, another benefit of continuous catheter techniques that may be less applicable to the sports medicine patient but significant for other orthopedic patient populations includes sympathectomy following digit implantation.[37–39] Finger and toe reimplantation may benefit from continuous infusions that allow for sympathectomy and improved blood flow to the transplanted limb.

CPNBs have been used in treating patients with phantom limb pain and complex regional pain syndrome (CRPS). The reduction of chronic pain following surgeries is another potential benefit of CPNBs. There have been some encouraging data in patients undergoing TKA demonstrating that continuous catheter techniques may reduce chronic pain in patients up to 6 months after surgery.[25] With a significant number of patients experiencing chronic pain after orthopedic surgeries, the potential to decrease this untoward outcome is critical. Although every patient should be carefully reviewed for the risks and benefits of CPNBs, there is mounting evidence that in addition to analgesic benefits, continuous catheters may also offer improved quality-of-life outcomes, functional outcomes, and cost savings to orthopedic patients.

CONSIDERATIONS FOR NERVE CATHETERS IN ORTHOPEDIC PATIENTS

A single injection nerve block can provide excellent analgesia for the orthopedic patient, but the continuous peripheral nerve catheter provides flexibility both in terms of duration of nerve block and density by controlling the dose and concentration of the local anesthetic infusate. With adjuvants added to local anesthetics, a single-injection nerve block can provide analgesia for up to 20 to 24 hours, but motor function and sensation cannot be assessed until resolution of the block. Nerve catheters allow the flexibility to lower the volume or concentration of the local anesthetic infusion to meet specific patient needs, thus also allowing for reduction of an initial local anesthetic bolus; this is important in situations in which assessment of motor function and sensation are needed such as with concern for compartment syndrome.[15]

Patient selection for CPNBs is critically important, especially in the ambulatory setting and in patients with comorbidities. Patients with renal or hepatic dysfunction are expected to have decreased clearance of local anesthetics and therefore should only receive a continuous nerve block catheter in a hospital or in a setting in which signs of local anesthetic toxicity can be directly monitored and treated.[40] Patients with renal or hepatic dysfunction should be carefully evaluated and potentially excluded from a home nerve catheter infusion. In addition, patients who are obese or those with cardiac and pulmonary disease, especially restrictive or obstructive lung disease pattern, should be carefully considered before placing an upper extremity nerve block catheter. These patients may be unable to compensate for the hypercarbia and/or hypoxia that can accompany an upper extremity nerve block because of phrenic nerve involvement and subsequent ipsilateral diaphragm paresis.[41] The preexisting pulmonary dysfunction of these patients and the potential for decreased hemidiaphragm excursion from the nerve block must be taken into account before both a single-injection nerve block and a peripheral nerve block catheter.

In the opioid-tolerant patient, managing acute postsurgical pain after orthopedic procedures can be challenging. Regional anesthesia with a peripheral nerve block catheter as part of a multimodal approach can reduce the opioid burden of these patients during the acute period when pain is most intense after surgery. Although regional anesthesia can reduce the need for additional opioid medications, baseline opioid requirements must be taken into account to prevent withdrawal symptoms.[42] On the other hand, opioid-sensitive and at-risk patients like those with obstructive sleep apnea are excellent patients to evaluate for a CPNB technique.

The preoperative placement of a continuous nerve catheter should also be considered in patients with CRPS undergoing orthopedic surgery. The development of CRPS after orthopedic surgery is not uncommon and estimated at 2.3% to 4% after arthroscopic knee surgery, 2.1% to 5% after carpal tunnel surgery, 13.6% after ankle surgery, 0.8% to 13% after TKA, 7% to 37% for wrist fractures, and 4.5% to 40% after fasciectomy for Dupuytren contracture.[43] It has been theorized that preoperative nerve blockade may reduce the recurrence of CRPS in patients with sympathetically mediated pain due to preoperative sympathetic blockade. Recommendations to reduce the development of CRPS type I in patients undergoing orthopedic surgery include adequate perioperative analgesia, reduction of operating time, limited use of tourniquet, and use of regional anesthesia.[44]

AMBULATORY CATHETER PUMPS

Ambulatory infusion pumps are categorized by their power source, and each device has its unique features and benefits. Pump preference usually depends on the clinical needs (ie, basal infusions, bolus dosing, and basal infusion + bolus capabilities) and logistic considerations. The 2 types of pumps available are electronic pumps and nonelectronic pumps. Nonelectronic pumps consist of spring-powered, vacuum-powered, and the more commonly used elastomeric pumps. The benefits of the electronic pumps are a more accurate and titratable basal infusion rate, patient-controlled bolus capabilities, and an adjustable bolus lockout period. The electronic pumps usually have an external reservoir of the local anesthetic, which allows for easy reservoir changes that can occur in an inpatient setting. Most electronic pumps are nondisposable and require returning the device for reuse, whereas the single-use reservoir cassettes are disposable.[9] The most recent and clinically impactful development of electronic pumps is the ability of the provider to remotely interact with the electronic pump via the Internet. This feature allows the health care provider to remotely control the pump based on text alert responses from the patient.[20]

The nonelectronic elastomeric pumps can be favored for simplicity in design, smaller size, lack of audible alarms, disposability, and also for allowing adjustments of infusion rates. Most elastomeric pumps have a fixed basal infusion rate set by the provider, and many do not have patient-controlled bolus capabilities; this often contributes to their decreased cost when compared with electronic pumps. These pumps also have an internal medication reservoir that does not allow replacement or refilling once the infusion has completed.[9] In more recent years, some of the available disposable pumps now allow for adjustable infusion rates and bolus capabilities (both patient initiated or at intervals set by the provider) with lockout periods similar to the electronic pumps.[20] Regardless of the pump power source, the ability to adjust the basal infusion is important to titrate local anesthetic administration in the case of an insensate extremity or unwanted side effects (ie, motor weakness). Adjusting the infusion rate is also helpful when analgesia is inadequate or when maximizing/minimizing infusion duration with a set local anesthetic reservoir volume. (**Fig. 1**)

CONSIDERATIONS FOR AMBULATORY NERVE CATHETERS

As ambulatory surgery grows in scope, more painful orthopedic surgery is being performed in ambulatory settings, including total shoulder arthroplasty, multiligament knee reconstruction, and ankle arthrodesis. The challenge presented to health care team members is to provide the patient with discharge readiness within hours of surgery while also prolonging postoperative analgesia after discharge home. As part of a multimodal analgesia regimen, a peripheral nerve block can provide optimal pain control and spare opioid-related side effects, whereas catheter placement can prolong postoperative analgesia at home.[45]

In addition to the traditional in-hospital setting, nerve block catheters have been successfully implemented in the ambulatory setting for both adult and pediatric patients using an at-home, portable infusion pump.[46] Patient selection is more stringent for an ambulatory nerve block catheter as opposed to a nerve block catheter being monitored in the hospital setting. The key to a safe at-home continuous nerve block catheter is proper patient selection, willingness of the patient to accept responsibility of the catheter and pump system, and appropriate patient education and resources. A discussion between the anesthesia provider and patient before catheter placement is essential to manage patient expectations and expected side effects. To safely discharge a patient with an at-home nerve catheter and infusion, the patient and their caregiver must be educated and able to comprehend the benefits and risks involved. The patient and caregiver should be given written and oral instructions on catheter care, infusion pump management, catheter removal, monitoring for signs of local anesthetic toxicity, and potential complications. The patient must also be educated on care of the insensate extremity and how the nerve block may affect their ambulation or physical therapy during the duration of the nerve blockade. For improved patient

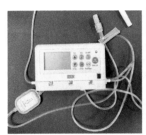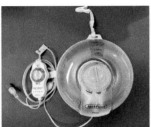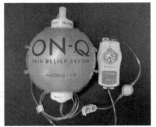

Fig. 1. Ambulatory infusion pumps: Nimbus PainPRO electronic pump (*left*). Arrow Auto-Fuser elastomeric pump (*middle*). Avanos ON-Q elastomeric pump (*right*).

satisfaction, expected occurrences such as local anesthetic leakage under catheter dressing and transition from surgical to analgesic block should be discussed.

Another critical aspect of a successful ambulatory catheter is 24-hour access to communication with an anesthesia provider for catheter- and pump-related concerns. Daily patient calls should be made from an experienced anesthesia provider to assess functioning of the catheter and any potential complications. Although there are well-published randomized controlled trial data on the analgesic benefits of ambulatory catheters, there are negligible data on optimal aspects of ambulatory infusions, such as requirement of a caregiver, patient oversight by provider, and catheter removal protocols.[9]

Nerve blocks can improve pain control and facilitate discharge from ambulatory settings after orthopedic procedures. The use of perineural catheters and portable infusions pumps can extend this analgesia for more than72 hours while the patient is at home, but preoperative planning, education, and proper patient selection is crucial for success. Exclusion criteria for at-home nerve catheters, such as patients with cognitive dysfunction, lack of reliability, lack of home support, baseline ambulation difficulty, and significant organ dysfunction should be taken into account before nerve catheter placement.[47,48]

COMPLICATIONS OF PERIPHERAL NERVE CATHETERS

In contrast to single-injection nerve blocks, complications unique to CPNBs must be considered. Peripheral nerve catheters carry the same risk as single-injection nerve blocks with regard to needle-induced and local anesthetic-induced complications. Major complications are rare, and minor complications are again similar to single-injection nerve blocks.[49] Failure of catheters is not uncommon, yet it is difficult to place a precise failure rate for all peripheral nerve catheters. Catheter failure can result from either primary (improper insertion) or secondary (catheter displacement, leakage, disconnection, or pump failure) factors. Given the wide variety of catheter locations, insertion techniques, securement devices/practices, and equipment differences, the published failure rates range from 1% to 50%.[50–52] However, given recent advancements in ultrasound technology and the decades of experience with peripheral nerve catheters, successful ambulatory and inpatient services have been implemented.

Benign complications are common yet are easily mitigated. Most common are leakage, dislodgement, and catheter obstruction. Most of these complications can be minimized by insertion technique, securement procedures, and patient education. Delivery device failure is rare, with the more common inadvertent pause, catheter kinking, and disconnections being amenable to patient and staff education.

Bleeding and hematoma formation is quite rare in the patient without coagulopathy. Even patients with bleeding diathesis or on anticoagulation can receive peripheral nerve catheters, but patient education is important in patients at higher risk of bleeding. Regarding superficial peripheral nerve blocks (most blocks performed for orthopedic surgery), national guidelines simply suggest the clinician consider the site, compressibility, vascularity, and consequences of bleeding should it occur at the chosen block site. Thus, it would be prudent for a practitioner to consider avoiding an interscalene catheter for a patient with a propensity to bleed.

When performing any peripheral nerve block, one should always consider the total dose of local anesthetic to avoid a potentially deadly incidence of local anesthetic systemic toxicity (LAST). The incidence of severe LAST tends to be associated with bolus dosing either upon initial placement or subsequent boluses.[53] Regarding continuous nerve blocks, about 15% of LAST cases occur in patients with continuous nerve catheters and typically present between days 1 to 4 of infusion. For this reason, it is critical that patients and families receive education about the symptoms of LAST and are instructed on how to stop the infusion and receive medical help. Of course, patient selection is key because those with decreased metabolism of local anesthetics will be at inherently higher risk including those with liver disease and neonates.[53]

With regard to neurologic injury, it is difficult to determine if continuous catheter techniques increase the incidence of neurologic injury. Whether indwelling catheters and prolonged infusions increase inflammatory neurotoxic effects of local anesthetics is still unresolved. All peripheral nerve blocks are associated with an inherent risk of neurologic injury; however, there has been some data to suggest an elevated risk of postoperative neurologic symptoms (PONS) with continuous nerve catheters when compared with single-injection nerve blocks. A study of 12,668 peripheral nerve blocks reported risk of PONS presenting past 6 months to be slightly elevated when compared with single-shot nerve blocks (0.24% versus 0.07%; $P = .08$).[54] However, it is difficult to know the true significance of this reported increase given they come from a retrospective review of a nonrandomized cohort. Two prospective studies by Fredrickson and colleagues[55,56] incorporated more than 2500 peripheral nerve catheters. The incidence of PONS was reported to be 4.9% to 5.3% resolving by 6 months and only 0.3% to 0.7% resolving by 11 months.[55,56] This reported rate of PONS is closer to the reported rates by most studies of peripheral nerve catheters and single-injection nerve blocks. Of course the rates will vary by nerve block site. When discussing neurologic injury, one must always consider the many benefits of the peripheral nerve block such as decreased pain and suffering, often improved surgical outcomes, and accelerated rehabilitation.

In the United States, the length of time that catheters may be left in place has not been standardized. The main concern with prolonged indwelling peripheral nerve catheters is the risk of catheter-related infection. A prospective multicenter study showed that the probability of peripheral infection-free catheter use was 99% at day 4 of catheter duration, 96% at day 7, and 73% at day 15.[47] The presence of diabetes and obesity elevate one's risk of catheter-related infection.[57–59] Abscess formation is possible, although rare. Most infections, depending on severity, resolve either spontaneously or with the addition of oral antibiotics. Infection requiring surgical intervention is quite rare. Nevertheless, it is imperative that patients with peripheral nerve catheters are routinely monitored; this can be achieved by an inpatient pain service when patients are admitted or through telephone communication with the ambulatory patient discharged home.

SUMMARY

Patients undergoing painful orthopedic surgery in the hospital or ambulatory setting should be screened for appropriateness and considered for a CPNB. In addition to prolongation of analgesia, the additional benefits of improved pain scores, decreased narcotic use, decreased opioid side effects, improved sleep, and improved patient satisfaction make CPNBs an important modality for postoperative pain control. With the growing scope of orthopedic surgery in the ambulatory setting, CPNBs can help facilitate discharge-readiness while providing cost-effective quality care. Careful consideration should be taken during patient selection for CPNBs based on medical comorbidities and ability to manage the ambulatory catheter and pump system. Last, it is essential to provide thorough patient/caregiver education and have experienced anesthesia providers available for communication regarding any side effects or potential complications.

DISCLOSURE

The authors have nothing to disclose.

REFERENCES

1. Ansbro F. A method of continuous brachial plexus block. Am J Surg 1946;71: 716–22.
2. Sarnoff S, Sarnoff L. Prolonged peripheral nerve block by means of indwelling plastic catheter; treatment of hiccup; note on the electrical localization of peripheral nerve. Anesthesiology 1951;12(3):270–5.
3. Dao T, Amaro-Driedger D, Mehta J. Successful treatment of Raynaud's syndrome in a lupus patient with continuous bilateral popliteal sciatic nerve blocks: a case report. Local Reg Anesth 2016;9:35–7.
4. Manriquez RG, Pallares V. Continuous brachial plexus block for prolonged sympathectomy and control of pain. Anesth Analg 1978;57(1):128–30.
5. Berger A, Tizian C, Zenz M. Continuous plexus blockade for improved circulation in microvascular surgery. Ann Plast Surg 1985;14(1):16–9.
6. Cheeley LN. Treatment of peripheral embolism by continuous sciatic nerve block. Curr Res Anesth Analg 1952;31(3):211–2.
7. Dadure C, Motais F, Ricard C, et al. Continuous peripheral nerve blocks at home for treatment of recurrent complex regional pain syndrome I in children. Anesthesiology 2005;102(2):387–91.
8. Ilfeld BM, Moeller-Bertram T, Hanling SR, et al. Treating intractable phantom limb pain with ambulatory continuous peripheral nerve blocks: a pilot study. Pain Med 2013;14(6):935–42.
9. Ilfeld BM. Continuous peripheral nerve blocks: a review of the published evidence. Anesth Analg 2011;113(4):904–25.
10. Borgeat A, Tewes E, Biasca N, et al. Patient-controlled interscalene analgesia with ropivacaine after major shoulder surgery: PCIA vs PCA. Br J Anaesth 1998;81(4):603–5.
11. Capdevila X, Pirat P, Bringuier S, et al. Continuous peripheral nerve blocks in hospital wards after orthopedic surgery: a multicenter prospective analysis of the quality of postoperative analgesia and complications in 1,416 patients. Anesthesiology 2005;103(5):1035–45.
12. Capdevila X, Dadure C, Bringuier S, et al. Effect of patient-controlled perineural analgesia on rehabilitation and pain after ambulatory orthopedic surgery: a multicenter randomized trial. Anesthesiology 2006;105(3):566–73.
13. Nikolajsen L, Brandsborg B, Lucht U, et al. Chronic pain following total hip arthroplasty: a nationwide questionnaire study. Acta Anaesthesiol Scand 2006;50(4): 495–500.
14. Puolakka PA, Rorarius MG, Roviola M, et al. Persistent pain following knee arthroplasty. Eur J Anaesthesiol 2010;27(5):455–60.
15. Aguirre J, Del Moral A, Cobo I, et al. The role of continuous peripheral nerve blocks. Anesthesiol Res Pract 2012;2012:560879.
16. Capdevila X, Bringuier S, Borgeat A, et al. Infectious Risk of Continuous Peripheral Nerve Blocks. Anesthesiology 2009;110(1):182–8.
17. Nicholson T, Maltenfort M, Getz C, et al. Multimodal Pain Management Protocol Versus Patient Controlled Narcotic Analgesia for Postoperative Pain Control after Shoulder Arthroplasty. Arch Bone Jt Surg 2018;6(3):196–202.
18. Kolarczyk LM, Williams BA. Transient heat hyperalgesia during resolution of ropivacaine sciatic nerve block in the rat. Reg Anesth Pain Med 2011;36(3):220–4.

19. Truini A. A Review of Neuropathic Pain: From Diagnostic Tests to Mechanisms. Pain Ther 2017;6(Suppl 1):5–9.
20. Ilfeld BM. Continuous Peripheral Nerve Blocks: An Update of the Published Evidence and Comparison With Novel, Alternative Analgesic Modalities. Anesth Analg 2017;124(1):308–35.
21. Sunderland S, Yarnold CH, Head SJ, et al. Regional Versus General Anesthesia and the Incidence of Unplanned Health Care Resource Utilization for Postoperative Pain After Wrist Fracture Surgery: Results From a Retrospective Quality Improvement Project. Reg Anesth Pain Med 2016;41(1):22–7.
22. Stathellis A, Fitz W, Schnurr C, et al. Periarticular injections with continuous perfusion of local anaesthetics provide better pain relief and better function compared to femoral and sciatic blocks after TKA: a randomized clinical trial. Knee Surg Sports Traumatol Arthrosc 2017;25(9):2702–7.
23. Ding DY, Manoli A 3rd, Galos DK, et al. Continuous Popliteal Sciatic Nerve Block Versus Single Injection Nerve Block for Ankle Fracture Surgery: A Prospective Randomized Comparative Trial. J Orthop Trauma 2015;29(9):393–8.
24. Sato K, Adachi T, Shirai N, et al. Continuous versus single-injection sciatic nerve block added to continuous femoral nerve block for analgesia after total knee arthroplasty: a prospective, randomized, double-blind study. Reg Anesth Pain Med 2014;39(3):225–9.
25. Sakai N, Inoue T, Kunugiza Y, et al. Continuous femoral versus epidural block for attainment of 120° knee flexion after total knee arthroplasty: a randomized controlled trial. J Arthroplasty 2013;28(5):807–14.
26. Peng L, Ren L, Qin P, et al. Continuous Femoral Nerve Block versus Intravenous Patient Controlled Analgesia for Knee Mobility and Long-Term Pain in Patients Receiving Total Knee Replacement: A Randomized Controlled Trial. Evid Based Complement Alternat Med 2014;2014:569107.
27. Lund J, Jenstrup MT, Jaeger P, et al. Continuous adductor-canal-blockade for adjuvant post-operative analgesia after major knee surgery: preliminary results. Acta Anaesthesiol Scand 2011;55(1):14–9.
28. Ilfeld BM, Hadzic A. Walking the tightrope after knee surgery: optimizing postoperative analgesia while minimizing quadriceps weakness. Anesthesiology 2013;118(2):248–50.
29. Jæger P, Zaric D, Fomsgaard JS, et al. Adductor canal block versus femoral nerve block for analgesia after total knee arthroplasty: a randomized, double-blind study. Reg Anesth Pain Med 2013;38(6):526–32.
30. Malhotra N, Madison SJ, Ward SR, et al. Continuous interscalene nerve block following adhesive capsulitis manipulation. Reg Anesth Pain Med 2013;38(2):171–2.
31. Salviz EA, Xu D, Frulla A, et al. Continuous interscalene block in patients having outpatient rotator cuff repair surgery: a prospective randomized trial. Anesth Analg 2013;117(6):1485–92.
32. Ilfeld BM, Enneking FK. Continuous peripheral nerve blocks at home: a review. Anesth Analg 2005;100(6):1822–33.
33. Ilfeld BM, Morey TE, Wang RD, et al. Continuous popliteal sciatic nerve block for postoperative pain control at home: a randomized, double-blinded, placebo-controlled study. Anesthesiology 2002;97(4):959–65.
34. Ilfeld BM, Morey TE, Enneking FK. Continuous infraclavicular brachial plexus block for postoperative pain control at home: a randomized, double-blinded, placebo-controlled study. Anesthesiology 2002;96(6):1297–304.

35. Shah NA, Jain NP. Is continuous adductor canal block better than continuous femoral nerve block after total knee arthroplasty? Effect on ambulation ability, early functional recovery and pain control: a randomized controlled trial. J Arthroplasty 2014;29(11):2224–9.
36. Cruz Eng H, Riazi S, Veillette C, et al. An Expedited Care Pathway with Ambulatory Brachial Plexus Analgesia Is a Cost-effective Alternative to Standard Inpatient Care after Complex Arthroscopic Elbow Surgery: A Randomized, Single-blinded Study. Anesthesiology 2015;123(6):1256–66.
37. Saporito A, Sturini E, Borgeat A, et al. The effect of continuous popliteal sciatic nerve block on unplanned postoperative visits and readmissions after foot surgery–a randomised, controlled study comparing day-care and inpatient management. Anaesthesia 2014;69(11):1197–205.
38. Su HH, Lui PW, Yu CL, et al. The effects of continuous axillary brachial plexus block with ropivacaine infusion on skin temperature and survival of crushed fingers after microsurgical replantation. Chang Gung Med J 2005;28(8):567–74.
39. Lang RS, Gorantla VS, Esper S, et al. Anesthetic management in upper extremity transplantation: the Pittsburgh experience. Anesth Analg 2012;115(3):678–88.
40. Denson DD, Raj PP, Saldahna F, et al. Continuous perineural infusion of bupivacaine for prolonged analgesia: pharmacokinetic considerations. Int J Clin Pharmacol Ther Toxicol 1983;21(12):591–7.
41. Borgeat A, Perschak H, Bird P, et al. Patient-controlled interscalene analgesia with ropivacaine 0.2% versus patient-controlled intravenous analgesia after major shoulder surgery: effects on diaphragmatic and respiratory function. Anesthesiology 2000;92(1):102–8.
42. Coluzzi F, Bifulco F, Cuomo A, et al. The challenge of perioperative pain management in opioid-tolerant patients. Ther Clin Risk Manag 2017;13:1163–73.
43. Reuben S, Warltier D. Preventing the Development of Complex Regional Pain Syndrome after Surgery. Anesthesiology 2004;101(5):1215–24.
44. Sumitani M, Yasunaga H, Uchida K, et al. Perioperative factors affecting the occurrence of acute complex regional pain syndrome following limb bone fracture surgery: data from the Japanese Diagnosis Procedure Combination database. Rheumatology (Oxford) 2014;53(7):1186–93.
45. Klein S, Evans H, Nielsen K, et al. Peripheral Nerve Block Techniques for Ambulatory Surgery. Anesth Analgesia 2005;1663–76.
46. Ganesh A, Rose J, Wells L, et al. Continuous Peripheral Nerve Blockade for Inpatient and Outpatient Postoperative Analgesia in Children. Anesth Analgesia 2007;105(5):1234–42.
47. Greengrass RA, Nielsen KC. Management of peripheral nerve block catheters at home. Int Anesthesiol Clin 2005;43(3):79–87.
48. Bomberg H, Bayer I, Wagenpfeil S, et al. Prolonged Catheter Use and Infection in Regional Anesthesia: A Retrospective Registry Analysis. Anesthesiology 2018;128(4):764–73.
49. Borgeat A, Ekatodramis G, Kalberer F, et al. Acute and nonacute complications associated with interscalene block and shoulder surgery: a prospective study. Anesthesiology 2001;95(4):875–80.
50. Neuburger M, Breitbarth J, Reisig F, et al. Komplikationen bei peripherer Katheterregionalanästhesie Untersuchungsergebnisse anhand von 3,491 Kathetern [Complications and adverse events in continuous peripheral regional anesthesia Results of investigations on 3,491 catheters]. Anaesthesist 2006;55(1):33–40.
51. Ilfeld BM, Morey TE, Wright TW, et al. Continuous interscalene brachial plexus block for postoperative pain control at home: a randomized, double-blinded,

placebo-controlled study. Anesth Analg 2003;96(4). https://doi.org/10.1213/01.ane.0000049824.51036.ef.

52. Ganapathy S, Wasserman RA, Watson JT, et al. Modified continuous femoral three-in-one block for postoperative pain after total knee arthroplasty. Anesth Analg 1999;89(5):1197–202.

53. Walker BJ, Long JB, Sathyamoorthy M, et al. Complications in Pediatric Regional Anesthesia: An Analysis of More than 100,000 Blocks from the Pediatric Regional Anesthesia Network. Anesthesiology 2018;129(4):721–32.

54. Sites BD, Taenzer AH, Herrick MD, et al. Incidence of local anesthetic systemic toxicity and postoperative neurologic symptoms associated with 12,668 ultrasound-guided nerve blocks: an analysis from a prospective clinical registry. Reg Anesth Pain Med 2012;37(5):478–82.

55. Fredrickson MJ, Leightley P, Wong A, et al. An analysis of 1505 consecutive patients receiving continuous interscalene analgesia at home: a multicentre prospective safety study. Anaesthesia 2016;71(4):373–9.

56. Fredrickson MJ, Kilfoyle DH. Neurological complication analysis of 1000 ultrasound guided peripheral nerve blocks for elective orthopaedic surgery: a prospective study. Anaesthesia 2009;64(8):836–44.

57. Bomberg H, Kubulus C, List F, et al. Diabetes: a risk factor for catheter-associated infections. Reg Anesth Pain Med 2015;40(1):16–21.

58. Bomberg H, Albert N, Schmitt K, et al. Obesity in regional anesthesia–a risk factor for peripheral catheter-related infections. Acta Anaesthesiol Scand 2015;59(8):1038–48.

59. Neal JM, Barrington MJ, Fettiplace MR, et al. The Third American Society of Regional Anesthesia and Pain Medicine Practice Advisory on Local Anesthetic Systemic Toxicity: Executive Summary 2017. Reg Anesth Pain Med 2018;43(2):113–23.

Regional Anesthesia Complications and Contraindications

Danial Shams, MD, Kaylyn Sachse, MD, Nicholas Statzer, MD,
Rajnish K. Gupta, MD*

KEYWORDS

- Nerve injury • Hematoma • Rebound pain • Regional anesthesia
- Neuraxial anesthesia

KEY POINTS

- While regional anesthesia brings with it a host of benefits, there are still risks involved with performing neuraxial and regional nerve blocks. Complications with regional anesthesia fall within 4 broad categories: block failure, bleeding/hematoma, neurologic injury, and local anesthetic toxicity (LAST).
- Block failure and rebound pain may undermine the benefits of regional anesthesia if steps are not taken to mitigate their risk. However, with diligence and the use of continuous nerve catheters/nerve block adjuncts, these risks may be minimized.
- Bleeding and hematoma formation are a risk with any regional technique. By identifying the appropriate patient factors and using techniques that have lower bleeding possibilities, the risk of significant or dangerous bleeding can be reduced.
- The risk of long-term neurologic injury can be categorized using the epidemiologic triangle. Through the recognition of patient and technique risk factors and by the utilization of appropriate monitoring, the risk of neurologic injury can be lessened.
- Local anesthetic systemic toxicity (LAST) can cause complete neurologic and cardiac collapse. Prompt recognition and treatment can minimize patient harm and improve outcomes.

INTRODUCTION

As an increasing number of orthopedic surgeries move from inpatient to outpatient settings, changes within anesthetic practices need to follow.[1] In ambulatory surgery, decreasing length of stay in the postanesthesia care unit (PACU) is a strong financial motivator and thus identifying the causes of increased length of stay become of utmost importance. Various studies have identified multiple factors associated with

Department of Anesthesiology, Vanderbilt University Medical Center, 1301 Medical Center Drive, 4648 TVC, Nashville, TN 37232, USA
* Corresponding author.
E-mail address: raj.gupta@vumc.org
Twitter: @dr_rajgupta (R.K.G.)

Clin Sports Med 41 (2022) 329–343
https://doi.org/10.1016/j.csm.2021.11.006
0278-5919/22/© 2021 Elsevier Inc. All rights reserved.

delayed discharge, including type of surgery, excessive pain, and postoperative nausea and vomiting (PONV).[2] Regional anesthesia has a strong role in minimizing postoperative pain, decreasing narcotic use and PONV, and, therefore, speeding discharge times. However, as with any procedure, regional anesthesia has both benefits and risks. While the benefits may often outweigh the risks, it is important to identify what those complications and contraindications may be, which patient populations are at highest risk, and how to mitigate those risks to the greatest extent possible. When looking at overall closed claims within anesthesia, regional block-related claims were the most common (with chronic pain claims doubling acute pain claims), followed by respiratory events, cardiovascular events, and equipment-related events.[3] Despite this, overall significant anesthesia complication rates remain low and significant complications secondary to regional anesthesia follow this trend.

While a variety of different regional techniques exist, complications tend to fall within 4 broad categories: block failure, bleeding/hematoma, neurologic injury, and local anesthetic toxicity. These 4 categories and specifics of the complications will be discussed later in discussion.

BLOCK FAILURE

The definition of block failure depends on the situation. In most studies looking at block efficacy, a failed or unsuccessful block is defined as a block that is unable to be used as the sole surgical anesthetic, necessitating additional local supplementation on the field, sedation, or the conversion to general anesthesia. Using these terms, studies cite block failure as ranging from approximately 5% to 20% depending on the type of block being performed.[4] Importantly, these studies do not look at situations whereby the nerve block was originally intended for postoperative analgesia. Block failure as defined as inadequate postoperative analgesia would have a lower failure rate than blocks intended as the sole anesthetic, as a surgical block requires a much more complete and dense effect to be successful than a block that reduces postoperative pain. Factors associated with failed block include higher BMI, higher ASA (American Society of Anesthesia) physical status, female gender, and substance use history.[4,5] The adoption of ultrasound-guidance in place of landmark or nerve stimulator guidance has led to an increase in efficacy via decreased block failure rates, decreased time to perform blocks, faster onsets of blocks, increased duration of blocks, and a decrease in certain complications such as inadvertent vascular puncture.[6,7] The impact of a failed block includes exposure to additional sedation/general anesthesia, inherent block risks without the benefits of a successful block, and in one study resulted in longer surgical times and longer PACU length of stay.[5]

REBOUND PAIN

Rebound pain is a relatively sudden and severe increase in pain that was previously well controlled, corresponding with peripheral nerve block resolution.[8] A recently published retrospective study found that nearly half of patients at an ambulatory surgery center who had a peripheral nerve block as part of their anesthetic, experienced severe rebound pain. Risk factors for rebound pain include surgical procedures involving bone, younger patients and females.[9] Additionally, rebound pain after brachial plexus block for ambulatory wrist surgery has also been associated with an increased incidence of unplanned physician visits after PACU discharge.[10] Proposed steps to help mitigate the occurrence of rebound pain include placing continuous nerve catheters rather than single-shot peripheral nerve blocks, using additives to prolong the nerve block duration, educating patients regarding taking analgesics before complete block resolution, and using multimodal analgesics after the nerve block resolves.[11] Failure to take steps to mitigate rebound pain has the potential to undermine the beneficial effects of regional anesthesia in the perioperative setting.

BLEEDING/HEMATOMA
Regional Anesthesia in the Patient at rRisk of Bleeding

Regional anesthesia of any kind carries some inherent risk of inducing bleeding, particularly in a patient with preexisting bleeding diathesis (eg, thrombocytopenia, coagulation factor deficiency, renal dysfunction, etc.) or medically induced coagulation dysfunction. Although bleeding complications are incredibly rare, certain types of bleeding can lead to devastating complications. Specifically, bleeding in the vertebral (neuraxial) column can lead to permanent paralysis if not addressed within 8 to 12 hours.[12–14] While performing some deep peripheral nerve blocks, occult bleeding can go unrecognized initially leading to critical anemia and/or hypovolemic shock. As there is a wide variety of bleeding disorders and medications that must be considered before placing a regional anesthetic, the American Society of Regional Anesthesia and Pain Medicine (ASRA) publishes guidelines that provide a detailed review of a variety of bleeding conditions and medications of concern. With anticoagulation and antiplatelet medications, ASRA provides specific guidance regarding when to stop these medications before performing a procedure and when a medication can be restarted after a procedure is performed. Careful consideration of medication timing is critical with the continuous introduction and adoption of novel direct oral anticoagulants (DOACs) and antiplatelet medications.[13,15–17]

Neuraxial Bleeding/Hematoma

Vertebral column hematoma risk after central neuraxial block varies significantly depending on the type of procedure and the patient situation. Epidural and combined spinal-epidural (CSE) have inherently higher risks of hematoma formation due to the larger needles used. Spinal anesthesia typically has a lower risk of bleeding. The risk for vertebral column hematoma in obstetric patients is extremely low with incidence reported at 1 in 168,000.[12] Perioperative epidural or CSE procedures have a higher risk of developing a hematoma with published incidences between 1 and 2 in 20,000, approximately a 10-fold higher risk than in the obstetric population. Due to this lower risk of vertebral column hematoma and the significant medical advantages of regional anesthesia versus general anesthesia in obstetrics, the Society for Obstetric Anesthesia and Perinatology has released a variation on the ASRA guidelines for this specific subpopulation.[18] Risk factors for vertebral column hematoma include preexisting coagulopathy, anticoagulation medications, kidney dysfunction, increasing age, female gender, spinal abnormalities, larger needle size, osteoporosis, and multiple needle attempts.[19]

When a vertebral column hematoma is suspected, diagnosis and definitive surgical decompression are critical emergency. Patients may experience a variety of symptoms, including back/leg pain, variable sensory changes, paralysis, loss of bowel/bladder function, or loss of reflexes. Weakness, even when mild, outside of the expected distribution of an epidural (ie, lower extremity weakness with a high thoracic epidural) can be one of the first presenting symptoms. Neurologic recovery can exceed 80% when spinal decompression is performed within 8 to 12 hours after the onset of hematoma. However, delay of surgical decompression beyond 12 hours from the onset of neurologic symptoms reduces the chance of meaningful neurologic recovery to less than 30%.[20] Diagnosis requires a rapid contrast magnetic resonance imaging (MRI) of the region of the spine whereby the epidural was performed and urgent coagulation laboratories (platelets, prothrombin time, partial thromboplastin time). Computerized tomography (CT) scans are typically inadequate to determine the extent of spinal cord compromise. Simultaneous surgical consultation and preparation of an operating room for epidural decompression are the treatments of choice.

Deep Peripheral Nerve Block Bleeding

ASRA makes a distinction in its guidelines between peripheral nerve blocks and neuraxial procedures as the risk of bleeding in the vertebral column can be so devastating. The incidence of major bleeding complications related to peripheral nerve blocks is extremely rare but also ill-defined and based on a series of case reports.[12,13] In one review of 6 cohort studies, an incidence of 0.67% [95%CI: 0.51%-0.83%] of bleeding complications was detected in patients chronically treated with antiplatelet and/or anticoagulation medications who received a peripheral nerve block (**Fig. 1**).[21] In addition, ASRA makes a distinction between superficial peripheral nerve blocks and deep peripheral nerve blocks. Although there is no specific categorization from ASRA of deep and superficial blocks, attempts have been made by experts in the field to develop a consensus summary of the level of bleeding risk associated with different blocks (**Table 1**).[22] Generally speaking, deep blocks include those that are located at noncompressible regions, are in the proximity of large vessels, in areas whereby neurologic symptoms may be delayed despite bleeding, in regions whereby occult bleeding can be significant, or are in the proximity of the spinal cord.[21,22] It is recommended that when practitioners are performing deep blocks, they use the same conservative guidelines that ASRA recommends for neuraxial blocks as bleeding in these

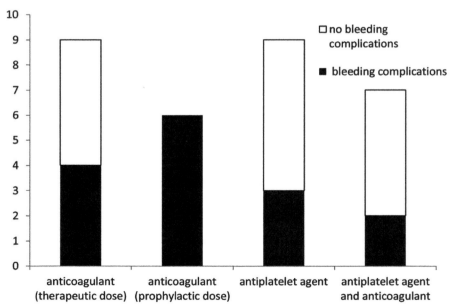

Fig. 1. Type and dose of anticlotting drugs, and incidence of bleeding complications in 31 patients identified in 18 reports. (*From*: Joubert, F. et al. Bleeding complications following peripheral regional anesthesia in patients treated with anticoagulants or antiplatelet agents: A systematic review. Anaesth Crit Care Pa 38, 507–516 (2019).)

Table 1
Consensus summary of the level of bleeding risk associated with different blocks

Body region	Blocks	Consensus	Grades[a]	Comments
Head and neck	Occipital nerve blocks	Low risk	III-B	No specific studies on bleeding risks; self-limited bleeding reported as secondary outcomes in 2 RCTs and 2 case series
	Superficial cervical plexus block (CPB)	Low risk	III-B	No specific studies on bleeding risks; no reports of bleeding from direct needle trauma in numerous studies involving superficial CPB
	Deep cervical plexus	High risk	III-B	No specific studies on bleeding risks; no reports of bleeding from direct needle trauma in numerous studies involving deep CPB
Above clavicle	Interscalene brachial plexus block	Intermediate risk	III-C	Incidental findings in an unrelated RCT or cohort were considered as a case report
	Supraclavicular brachial plexus block	Intermediate risk	III-C	Incidental findings in an unrelated RCT or cohort were considered as a case report
Below clavicle	Infraclavicular brachial plexus block	Intermediate risk	III-C	Incidental findings in an unrelated RCT or cohort were considered a case report
	Axillary brachial plexus block	Low risk	III-C	Incidental findings in an unrelated RCT or cohort were considered a case report
	Median, radial, ulnar nerve block	Low risk	IV-C	No specific data
Lumbar plexus	Lumbar plexus block	High risk	III-B	Multiple reports
	Femoral nerve block	Intermediate risk	III-C	Only one report
	Lateral femoral cutaneous nerve block	Low risk	IV-C	No specific data
	Suprainguinal fascia iliaca block	Intermediate risk	IV-C	No specific data
	Infrainguinal fascia iliaca block	Low risk	IV-C	No specific data
	Obturator nerve block	Intermediate risk	IV-C	No specific data
	Adductor canal nerve block	Intermediate risk	IV-C	No specific data

(continued on next page)

Table 1
(continued)

Body region	Blocks	Consensus	Grades[a]	Comments
Sacral plexus	Proximal sciatic nerve block (anterior, transgluteal, subgluteal)	Intermediate risk	IV-C	No specific data
	Popliteal sciatic nerve blocks	Intermediate risk	IV-C	No specific data
Ankle	Ankle block	Low risk	IV-C	No specific data
Interfascial plane	Rectus sheath	Intermediate risk	III-C	The highest evidence is from an RCT but downgraded because of the quality of the study
	Transversus abdominis (TAP) blocks	Intermediate risk	III-C	The highest evidence is from an observational study but downgraded because of the quality of the study
	TAP subcostal	Intermediate risk	IV-C	No specific data
	IIN/IHG	Intermediate risk	III-C	The highest evidence is from case reports
	Quadratus lumborum blocks	High risk	IV-C	No specific data
	Transversalis fascia block	Intermediate risk	IV-C	No specific data
	Erector spinae plane block	Low risk	IV-C	No specific data
	Pectoralis nerve (Pecs) 1	Intermediate risk	III-C	The highest evidence is from an RCT but downgraded because of the quality of the study
	Pectoralis nerve (Pecs) 2	Intermediate risk	IV-C	No specific data
	Serratus anterior plane block	Intermediate risk	IV-C	No specific data
Truncal	Paravertebral block	High risk	III-B	Several large and medium-sized case series, case reports, and incidental secondary outcome results from unrelated trials
	Intercostal block	Intermediate risk	III-C	No specific studies on bleeding risks; case reports of self-limited but occasionally significant bleeding outcomes

Abbreviations: IIN/IHG, ilioinguinal iliohypogastric nerve; RCT, randomized-controlled trial; TAP, transversus abdominis plane block.
[a] See **Table 2** for details of the grading system.
From: Tsui, B. C. H. et al. Practice advisory on the bleeding risks for peripheral nerve and interfascial plane blockade: evidence review and expert consensus. Can J Anesthesia J Can D'anesthésie 66, 1356–1384 (2019).

areas can lead to hematoma formation resulting in neurologic injury which may be delayed or significant, hematomas which may require surgical decompression, or even hemodynamic collapse when bleeding goes unrecognized.[13,21] Examples of deep peripheral nerve blocks include lumbar plexus blocks and paravertebral blocks. There are some blocks, such as erector spinae block, supraclavicular block, and quadratus lumborum block that have instigated ongoing debate regarding bleeding risk and how conservative regional anesthesiologists should be regarding anticoagulation and bleeding diatheses.

Superficial Peripheral Nerve Block Bleeding

Superficial peripheral nerve blocks are those blocks whereby bleeding can be easily recognized due to surface bleeding or bruising and whereby the compression of the region is an effective means of controlling the bleeding until definitive hemostasis can be established. Examples of superficial nerve blocks include interscalene block, axillary block, femoral nerve block, and popliteal sciatic nerve block. When performing superficial peripheral nerve blocks, ASRA only recommends that the practitioner take the clinical situation into consideration and typically does not provide specific guidance on holding medications before procedures due to the overall low risk.

Fascial Plane Blocks and Bleeding

In the last decade, a variety of fascial plane blocks has been described and become widely used. These blocks are typically performed in the fascial plane between muscle layers, use large volumes of local anesthetic to block nerves passing through those layers, and do not directly target specific nerves themselves. Many of these blocks are superficial and compressible (eg, TAP block, PECS block, rectus sheath block). A few are deeper and may vary in their bleeding risk depending on the patient's body habitus (eg, erector spinae block, quadratus lumborum block). ASRA does not currently provide guidance on the risk of bleeding surrounding fascial plane blocks and there is ongoing debate as to which of these blocks should be considered deep versus superficial.[23–26]

NEUROLOGIC INJURY

Long-term neurologic injuries (>6 months) with regional anesthesia are a feared yet rare complication, both with neuraxial and peripheral nerve blocks (PNB), with prospective studies finding they occur in approximately 2 to 4 in 10,000 blocks.[27–30] Transient neurologic symptoms, on the other hand, occur at a higher frequency, yet often resolve within 3 to 6 months of the injury.[28] However, neurologic injuries can be debilitating and devastating when they do occur. Various etiologies of neurologic injury have been described, including trauma secondary to the block needle, pressure injury,[31] local anesthetic or adjuvant toxicity, and ischemia, not to mention other factors such as patient characteristics and surgical type. Due to the multiplicity of factors in play when it comes to neurologic injury and nerve blocks, *Complications of Regional Anesthesia* notes that it may be best to think of it "using the same epidemiologic principles of disease causation." In this vein, it should be thought of using the "epidemiologic triangle," which encompasses causative agents (such as mechanical or chemical injury), host factors (such as surgical and patient elements), and environmental influences (such as safe practices and methods to detect intraneural injection).[30] Thus, eliminating as many components of this triangle as possible may lead to prevention or at least minimization or risk of complications. These are outlined separately later in discussion.

Host Factors

Preexisting neuropathy
Although there is no significant evidence to support that preexisting neurologic dysfunction leads to increased vulnerability to further neurologic damage, there have been many case reports indicating this.[32] In these cases, it is possible a "two-hit" hypothesis or double crush syndrome may be applicable. Thus, it is advisable to treat patients with known neuropathic disease, such as those with prior neurologic injury, diabetic neuropathy, peripheral vascular disease (PVD), chemotherapy-induced peripheral neuropathy (CIPN), or any number of disease processes with neurologic involvement (such as multiple sclerosis, lupus, etc.), with additional care and decide on a case-by-case basis whether a PNB is appropriate.

Surgical elements
Cases with trauma, prolonged tourniquet time, or high levels of neural stretch can be associated with increased likelihood of nerve injuries. Neuropraxias have been previously reported across multiple orthopedic surgeries, including arthroscopic shoulder surgery (16%–30%),[33] total shoulder arthroplasty (0.8%–4.3%),[34] total knee arthroplasty (0.3%–1.3%),[35] and total hip arthroplasty (0.6%–3.7%).[33,36]

Causative Agents

Needle trauma
In clinical studies, it has been demonstrated that the presence of paresthesias during PNBs can increase the risk of postoperative neurologic symptoms.[29] Additionally, merely the shape or design of needles can also impact the risk of neuropraxias. In a cadaver study, Sala-Blanch et al. demonstrated that long-bevel needles (30°) introduce a higher risk of intrafascicular injection than short-bevel needles (15°). However, regardless of the type of needle used, the risk of intrafascicular injection was believed to be low than interfascicular injection, which may not lead to nerve injury.[37]

Pressure injury
Higher injection pressures at the outset of injection may indicate a needle is intraneural; this can lead to fascicular injury and, consequently, neurologic deficits.[31] Thus, it can be hypothesized that the avoidance of excessive injection pressures can decrease the risk of neurologic injury.

Environmental Influences

Ultrasound versus nerve stimulation
Retrospective studies show no difference in neurologic complications between nerve stimulation and ultrasound-guidance. However, this does not mean ultrasound-guidance has no place in PNBs as it has been shown to decrease cases of local anesthetic toxicity, increase block efficacy, decrease block failure rates, decrease time to block completion, speed up to block onset, and increase their duration compared with nerve stimulation.[7,38,39]

Injection pressure monitoring
As mentioned above, high-pressure injections have been histologically shown to cause likely fascicular injury.[31] Additionally, studies have shown that experience does not help providers determine whether pressures are high by syringe feel only.[40] Therefore, techniques such as compressed air injection technique (CAIT)[41] or pressure measurement devices may have a role in helping to minimize the risk of intrafascicular injection and consequent neurologic injury.

Prevention and Management

As evidenced above, neurologic injuries in the setting of regional anesthesia are multifactorial and complex in origin. Using the idea of the "epidemiologic triangle" can assist providers in minimizing risk factors from some or all the aspects of the triangle, thus overall decreasing the risk of long-term neurologic harm to patients. Via risk stratification, at-risk patients can be identified, and the increased risk of neurologic injury can be discussed with the patients. Open communication during the procedure itself will allow providers to hopefully decrease the risk of paresthesias. Appropriate monitoring techniques will help to reduce the possibility of intraneural or intrafascicular injections. Follow-up and early referral for those with evidence of iatrogenic injury can increase the possibility of recovery and minimize long-term disability.

LOCAL ANESTHETIC SYSTEMIC TOXICITY
Overview of LAST

Local anesthetic systemic toxicity (LAST) is a well-documented regional anesthetic complication. LAST is a complex syndrome resulting from toxic effects of local anesthetics in tissues sensitive to their effects, primarily the central nervous system (CNS) and cardiac conduction systems. The observed clinical effects of LAST vary widely, ranging from mild CNS excitement such as tinnitus and circumoral numbness, to severe, life-threatening effects including seizures, arrhythmias, and/or cardiovascular collapse. Prompt diagnosis and treatment are essential to avoid severe complications resulting from LAST. ASRA has published practice guidelines that guide the identification and treatment of LAST.[42]

Mechanisms of Local Anesthetic Toxicity

Toxic effects of local anesthetics result when excessive concentrations accumulate in tissues sensitive to their effects and intolerant of hypoxemia such as the cardiovascular and central nervous systems.

Drug and Dose

Dose and drug administered may influence the severity of symptoms (**Table 2**). In general, CNS symptoms occur at lower plasma concentrations than cardiovascular (CV) symptoms of LAST. The difference in plasma concentration required to cause seizures compared with the concentration at which cardiovascular collapse occurs is termed the CV/CNS ratio.[43] Bupivacaine, in particular, has been associated with a decreased CV/CNS ratio and thus has a smaller therapeutic window compared with other amide local anesthetics. This difference may be explained by bupivacaine's increased binding affinity to cardiac voltage-gated sodium channels. Bupivacaine has also been shown to have greater impact in increasing atrial-ventricular-conduction time and greater cardiodepressant effects than ropivacaine.[44,45]

Cardiovascular Toxicity

The mechanism of cardiovascular dysfunction is complex. Indeed, the exact mechanism of direct cardiovascular toxicity is not fully understood. In part, decreased AV-node activity and conduction blockade within the His-Purkinje system, evidenced by widening QRS complexes, and resulting dysrhythmia may be observed.[46,47] Any newly observed dysrhythmia should be suspected as early toxicity and should trigger cessation of LA administration.

Central Nervous System Toxicity

CNS toxicity follows a two-phase pattern; an initial excitatory phase is followed by a depressive phase as local anesthetic concentrations are increased. The excitatory phase occurs as inhibitory interneurons are blocked at lower local anesthetic concentrations,[48] leading to tinnitus, circumoral numbness, or metallic taste perception, followed by psychomotor agitation and eventual convulsion

Identification and Diagnosis of LAST

Presenting symptoms may vary widely and are dependent on several factors such as drug, dose, site of injection, and patient factors. As noted above, classic teaching describes a stepwise progression from CNS excitation (auditory changes, perioral numbness, agitation, and seizure), followed by CVS changes (EKG changes, hyper or hypotension, dysrhythmia, and eventual cardiovascular collapse). Fewer than 50% of cases follow this progression, with up to 24% presenting with CVS symptoms alone.[49] Additionally, the timing of LAST following injection may vary widely, from immediately following injection in the case of intravascular injection to hours later in the case of large-dose local infiltration, such as tumescent anesthesia.[50] Following LA injection, it is recommended to monitor patients for signs of LAST for at least 30 minutes.[51] Because of the heterogeneity of presenting symptoms, vigilance during and after procedures is essential to identifying and treating LAST.

Prevention Strategies

Prevention of LAST consists of preprocedure planning and preparation and intraprocedure avoidance of intravascular injection and careful calculations of maximal local anesthetic doses based on patient weight and comorbidities. Before a regional anesthetic procedure, patient factors that may increase predisposition to LAST should be identified. This may include low body weight or reduced muscle mass, cardiac conduction abnormalities, history of seizure, renal failure, pregnancy, and extremes of age. Maximum safe doses of local anesthetic should be calculated, drawing up no more than the allowable dose before the procedure. Minimum effective doses should be used whenever possible. Intraprocedure utilization of ultrasound-guidance has been associated with a 65% reduction in LAST events, due to improved ability to identify vascular structures.[52] Furthermore, ultrasound guidance allows increased precision of local anesthetic deposition, thus requiring lower volumes for effective block.[53–55] Careful aspiration before injection and observation for blood return should be performed. Injection of small aliquots (~5 mL) with intermittent aspiration is encouraged. **Table 2**

Table 2		
Maximum doses for common amide local anesthetics (single dose)		
		Maximum Dose	
LA Drug	Plain	With Epinephrine
Bupivacaine	2 mg/kg	3 mg/kg
Levobupivacaine	2 mg/kg	3 mg/kg
Ropivacaine	3 mg/kg	4 mg/kg
Lidocaine	5 mg/kg	7 mg/kg
Mepivacaine	5 mg/kg	7 mg/kg
Prilocaine	6 mg/kg	8 mg/kg

Treatment of Last

The 2018 ASRA Practice Guideline summarizes the key steps to managing a LAST event.[42] Lipid emulsion (20% lipid emulsion, *Intralipid*) therapy is central to the treatment of LAST. Lipid emulsion serves as a shuttle for LA molecules, drawing them away from highly perfused tissues to a depot in less perfused skeletal muscle. An initial bolus of 100 mL (>70 kg patient) or 1.5 mL/kg (<70 kg patient), followed by an infusion of 200 to 250 mL (>70 kg) or 0.25 mL/kg/min (<70 kg) over 15 to 20 minutes is recommended. This infusion should be maintained for 15 to 20 minutes after CVS stability has been achieved. Propofol is not an acceptable alternative to lipid emulsion. Other conditions such as hypoxemia, hypercapnia, and acidosis should be treated as they can worsen or prolong LAST. Benzodiazepines are preferred for seizure control, though succinylcholine may be used in refractory cases. If ACLS is required, resuscitation in LAST requires several alterations. Epinephrine dosing should be reduced (<1 mcg/kg). Typical code-dose epinephrine has been associated with worse outcomes in animal models due to a variety of mechanisms, including hyperlactatemia, acidosis, and impaired pulmonary exchange.[56–58] Vasopressin should be avoided. Calcium channel blockers and beta-antagonists are not recommended due to their potential to worsen conduction blockade. Amiodarone is the preferred agent to manage ventricular arrhythmias. Early notification of the nearest facility with ECMO capabilities should be considered due to the potential need for prolonged cardiopulmonary resuscitation.

DISCUSSION AND FUTURE DIRECTIONS

Neuraxial and peripheral nerve blocks provide patients with many benefits during the perioperative setting, but they are not performed without risk. Complications can range from relatively benign and short lived, such as small areas of temporary numbness, to severe and permanent, such as paralysis. Special consideration should be given to those patients identified as high risk for complications (preexisting nerve injury, coagulopathy, etc.) to help mitigate complications. Just as the use of ultrasound has revolutionized peripheral block placement over the last 20 years, future developments could have large impacts on the safety and efficacy of regional anesthesia. For example, devices with the ability to monitor injection pressures may become more widely available and the standardization of their use may reduce the incidence of unintended nerve injury. Additionally, as new antiplatelet and anticoagulation medications are used in clinical practice, further guidelines regarding the timing of their use in relation to neuraxial block placement will need to be developed.

CLINICS CARE POINTS

- Regional anesthesia, in the hands of an experienced provider, is safe, beneficial, and has a strong role to play in ambulatory surgeries. While the rate of complications may be low, it behooves providers to know what these may be and how to avoid them.

- Block failure is a real possibility, particularly when a block is used as the primary anesthetic; however, when used for postoperative analgesia, the rate of "failure" may be lower. Rebound pain is possible with any regional anesthetic but the effects can be mitigated by using peripheral nerve catheters or nerve block adjuncts to extend the duration of blocks. Good patient education with expectation management and the use of multimodal analgesics are essential.

- While the risk of bleeding and hematoma formation are present with any regional anesthetic procedure, correct identification of patient risk factors and utilization of appropriate techniques will allow providers to hopefully avoid any significant deleterious outcomes.

- The risk of long-term neurologic injury is low but very feared among both providers and patients. By avoiding intrafascicular injection, monitoring injection pressures, and possibly avoiding blocks in high-risk patients, poor outcomes can be reduced.
- Local anesthetic systemic toxicity (LAST) is a known risk for any regional anesthesia procedure, but the risk of acute LAST has decreased with the advent of ultrasound-guided regional blocks. Prompt recognition of early toxicity symptoms and early implementation of treatment (primarily the use of intralipid) can help minimize patient harm.

DISCLOSURE

Dr. R.K. Gupta is on the Board of Directors of the American Society of Regional Anesthesia and Pain Medicine (ASRA Pain Medicine). He is the lead developer of the ASRA Coags, LAST, and Timeout apps for which he has received royalties in the past. Dr. R.K. Gupta also serves as an Associate Editor for the journal Regional Anesthesia and Pain Medicine. Dr. R.K. Gupta receives research funding from the NIH (R01 DA050334-01A1).

REFERENCES

1. Cozowicz C, Poeran J, Memtsoudis SG. Epidemiology, trends, and disparities in regional anaesthesia for orthopaedic surgery. Bja Br J Anaesth 2015; 115(suppl_2):ii57–67.
2. Chung F, Mezei G. Factors contributing to a prolonged stay after ambulatory surgery. Anesth Analg 1999;89(6):1352.
3. Metzner J, Posner KL, Lam MS, et al. Closed claims' analysis. Best Pract Res Clin Anaesthesiol 2011;25(2):263–76.
4. Cotter JT, Nielsen KC, Guller U, et al. Increased body mass index and ASA physical status IV are risk factors for block failure in ambulatory surgery — an analysis of 9,342 blocks. Can J Anesth 2004;51(8):810.
5. Picard L, Belnou P, Debes C, et al. Impact of regional block failure in ambulatory hand surgery on patient management: a cohort study. J Clin Med 2020;9(8):2453.
6. Abrahams MS, Aziz MF, Fu RF, et al. Ultrasound guidance compared with electrical neurostimulation for peripheral nerve block: a systematic review and meta-analysis of randomized controlled trials. Bja Br J Anaesth 2009;102(3):408–17.
7. Schnabel A, Meyer-Frießem CH, Zahn PK, et al. Ultrasound compared with nerve stimulation guidance for peripheral nerve catheter placement: a meta-analysis of randomized controlled trials. Bja Br J Anaesth 2013;111(4):564–72.
8. Williams BA, Bottegal MT, Kentor ML, et al. Rebound pain scores as a function of femoral nerve block duration after anterior cruciate ligament reconstruction: retrospective analysis of a prospective, randomized clinical trial. Reg Anesth Pain Med 2007;32(3):186–92.
9. Barry GS, Bailey JG, Sardinha J, et al. Factors associated with rebound pain after peripheral nerve block for ambulatory surgery. Br J Anaesth 2021;126(4):862–71.
10. Sunderland S, Yarnold CH, Head SJ, et al. Regional versus general anesthesia and the incidence of unplanned health care resource utilization for postoperative pain after wrist fracture surgery. Region Anesth Pain M 2016;41(1):22–7.
11. Dada O, Zacarias AG, Ongaigui C, et al. Does rebound pain after peripheral nerve block for orthopedic surgery impact postoperative analgesia and opioid consumption? a narrative review. Int J Environ Res Pu 2019;16(18):3257.

12. Ashken T, West S. Regional anaesthesia in patients at risk of bleeding. Bja Educ 2021;21(3):84–94.
13. Horlocker TT, Vandermeuelen E, Kopp SL, et al. Regional anesthesia in the patient receiving antithrombotic or thrombolytic therapy. Region Anesth Pain M 2018;43(3):263–309.
14. Lee LA, Posner KL, Domino KB, et al. Injuries associated with regional anesthesia in the 1980s and 1990s. Anesthesiology 2004;101(1):143–52.
15. Kaye AD, Brunk AJ, Kaye AJ, et al. Regional anesthesia in patients on anticoagulation therapies—evidence-based recommendations. Curr Pain Headache R 2019;23(9):67.
16. Kai AM, Vadivelu N, Urman RD, et al. Perioperative considerations in the management of anticoagulation therapy for patients undergoing surgery. Curr Pain Headache R 2019;23(2):13.
17. Cappelleri G, Fanelli A. Use of direct oral anticoagulants with regional anesthesia in orthopedic patients. J Clin Anesth 2016;32:224–35.
18. Leffert L, Butwick A, Carvalho B, et al. The Society for Obstetric Anesthesia and Perinatology Consensus Statement on the Anesthetic Management of Pregnant and Postpartum Women Receiving Thromboprophylaxis or Higher Dose Anticoagulants. Anesth Analgesia 2018;126(3):928–44.
19. Liu H, Brown M, Sun L, et al. Complications and liability related to regional and neuraxial anesthesia. Best Pract Res Clin Anaesthesiol 2019;33(4):487–97.
20. Neal JM, Barrington MJ, Brull R, et al. The Second ASRA Practice Advisory on Neurologic Complications Associated With Regional Anesthesia and Pain Medicine. Region Anesth Pain M 2015;40(5):401–30.
21. Joubert F, Gillois P, Bouaziz H, et al. Bleeding complications following peripheral regional anaesthesia in patients treated with anticoagulants or antiplatelet agents: A systematic review. Anaesth Crit Care Pa 2019;38(5):507–16.
22. Tsui BCH, Kirkham K, Kwofie MK, et al. Practice advisory on the bleeding risks for peripheral nerve and interfascial plane blockade: evidence review and expert consensus. Can J Anesth J Can D'anesthésie. 2019;66(11):1356–84.
23. Galacho J, Veiga M, Ormonde L. Erector spinae plane block and altered hemostasis: is it a safe option? -a case series-. Korean J Anesthesiol 2020;73(5):445–9.
24. Salhotra R. Ultrasound-guided truncal/plane blocks: Are they safe in anticoagulated patients? J Anaesthesiol Clin Pharmacol 2020;36(1):118.
25. Tsui BCH, Fonseca A, Munshey F, et al. The erector spinae plane (ESP) block: A pooled review of 242 cases. J Clin Anesth 2019;53:29–34.
26. Adhikary SD, Prasad A, Soleimani B, et al. Continuous erector spinae plane block as an effective analgesic option in anticoagulated patients following left ventricular assist device implantation: A case series. J Cardiothor Vasc Anesth 2018; 33(4):1063–7.
27. Walker BJ, Long JB, Sathyamoorthy M, et al. Complications in pediatric regional anesthesia: an analysis of more than 100,000 blocks from the pediatric regional anesthesia network. Anesthesiology 2018;129(4):721–32.
28. Auroy Y, Benhamou D, Bargues L, et al. Major complications of regional anesthesia in France. Anesthesiology 2002;97(5):1274–80.
29. Fredrickson MJ, Kilfoyle DH. Neurological complication analysis of 1000 ultrasound guided peripheral nerve blocks for elective orthopaedic surgery: a prospective study. Anaesthesia 2009;64(8):836–44.
30. Finucane BT, Tsui BCH. Complications of regional anesthesia: Principles of safe practice in local and regional anesthesia. Third Edition. 2017.

31. Hadzic A, Dilberovic F, Shah S, et al. Combination of intraneural injection and high injection pressure leads to fascicular injury and neurologic deficits in dogs. Region Anesth Pain M 2004;29(5):417–23.
32. Blumenthal S, Borgeat A, Maurer K, et al. Preexisting subclinical neuropathy as a risk factor for nerve injury after continuous ropivacaine administration through a femoral nerve catheter. Anesthesiology 2006;105(5):1053–6.
33. Rodeo SA, Forster RA, Weiland AJ. Neurological complications due to arthroscopy. J Bone Jt Surg 1993;75(6):917–26.
34. Lädermann A, Lübbeke A, Mélis B, et al. Prevalence of neurologic lesions after total shoulder arthroplasty. J Bone Jt Surg 2011;93(14):1288–93.
35. Shetty T, Nguyen JT, Sasaki M, et al. Risk factors for acute nerve injury after total knee arthroplasty. Muscle Nerve 2018;57(6):946–50.
36. Hasija R, Kelly JJ, Shah NV, et al. Nerve injuries associated with total hip arthroplasty. J Clin Orthop Trauma 2018;9(1):81–6.
37. Sala-Blanch X, Ribalta T, Rivas E, et al. Structural injury to the human sciatic nerve after intraneural needle insertion. Region Anesth Pain M 2009;34(3):201–5.
38. Orebaugh SL, Kentor ML, Williams BA. Adverse outcomes associated with nerve stimulator–guided and ultrasound-guided peripheral nerve blocks by supervised trainees. Region Anesth Pain M 2012;37(6):577–82.
39. Orebaugh SL, Williams BA, Vallejo M, et al. Adverse outcomes associated with stimulator-based peripheral nerve blocks with versus without ultrasound visualization. Region Anesth Pain M 2009;34(3):251–5.
40. Theron PS, Mackay Z, Gonzalez JG, et al. An animal model of "syringe feel" during peripheral nerve block. Region Anesth Pain M 2009;34(4):330–2.
41. Tsui BCH, Knezevich MP, Pillay JJ. Reduced injection pressures using a compressed air injection technique (CAIT): an in vitro study. Region Anesth Pain M 2008;33(2):168–73.
42. Neal JM, Barrington MJ, Fettiplace MR, et al. The third american society of regional anesthesia and pain medicine practice advisory on local anesthetic systemic toxicity. Region Anesth Pain M 2018;43(2):113–23.
43. El-Boghdadly K, Chin KJ. Local anesthetic systemic toxicity: continuing professional development. Can J Anesth J Can D'anesthésie. 2016;63(3):330–49.
44. Graf BM, Abraham I, Eberbach N, et al. Differences in cardiotoxicity of bupivacaine and ropivacaine are the result of physicochemical and stereoselective properties. Anesthesiology 2002;96(6):1427–34.
45. Royse CF, Royse AG. The myocardial and vascular effects of bupivacaine, levobupivacaine, and ropivacaine using pressure volume loops. Anesth Analgesia 2005;101(3):679–87.
46. Coussaye JE de L, Eledjam J-J, Bruelle P, et al. Mechanisms of the putative cardioprotective effect of hexamethonium in anesthetized dogs given a large dose of bupivacaine. Anesthesiology 1994;80(3):595–605.
47. Butterworth JF. Models and mechanisms of local anesthetic cardiac toxicity. Region Anesth Pain M 2010;35(2):167–76.
48. Zink W, Graf BM. The toxicity of local anesthetics: the place of ropivacaine and levobupivacaine. Curr Opin Anaesthesiol 2008;21(5):645–50.
49. Gitman M, Barrington MJ. Local anesthetic systemic toxicity. Region Anesth Pain M 2018;43(2):124–30.
50. Vasques F, Behr AU, Weinberg G, et al. A review of local anesthetic systemic toxicity cases since publication of the american society of regional anesthesia recommendations. Region Anesth Pain M 2015;40(6):698–705.

51. Neal JM, Bernards CM, Butterworth JF, et al. ASRA practice advisory on local anesthetic systemic toxicity. Region Anesth Pain M 2010;35(2):152–61.
52. Barrington MJ, Kluger R. Ultrasound guidance reduces the risk of local anesthetic systemic toxicity following peripheral nerve blockade. Region Anesth Pain M 2013;38(4):289–99.
53. Latzke D, Marhofer P, Zeitlinger M, et al. Minimal local anaesthetic volumes for sciatic nerve block: evaluation of ED99 in volunteers. Bja Br J Anaesth 2010; 104(2):239–44.
54. O'Donnell BD, Iohom G. An estimation of the minimum effective anesthetic volume of 2% lidocaine in ultrasound-guided axillary brachial plexus block. Anesthesiology 2009;111(1):25–9.
55. Riazi S, Carmichael N, Awad I, et al. Effect of local anaesthetic volume (20 vs 5 ml) on the efficacy and respiratory consequences of ultrasound-guided interscalene brachial plexus block. Bja Br J Anaesth 2008;101(4):549–56.
56. Hiller DB, Gregorio GD, Ripper R, et al. Epinephrine impairs lipid resuscitation from bupivacaine overdose. Anesthesiology 2009;111(3):498–505.
57. Wang Q-G, Wu C, Xia Y, et al. Epinephrine deteriorates pulmonary gas exchange in a rat model of bupivacaine-induced cardiotoxicity. Region Anesth Pain M 2017; 42(3):342–50.
58. Weinberg GL, Gregorio GD, Ripper R, et al. Resuscitation with lipid versus epinephrine in a rat model of bupivacaine overdose. Anesthesiology 2008; 108(5):907–13.

A Look Forward and a Look Back

The Growing Role of ERAS Protocols in Orthopedic Surgery

Marissa Weber, MD[a],*, Melissa Chao, MD[b], Simrat Kaur, DO[c],
Bryant Tran, MD[c], Anis Dizdarevic, MD[b]

KEYWORDS

- ERAS • Multimodal analgesia • Ambulatory surgery • Orthopedic surgery
- Clinical pathways

KEY POINTS

- Enhanced Recovery after Surgery (ERAS) is a multidisciplinary, multimodal, protocol-based perioperative care model that aims to improve and expedite patient recovery after surgery
- ERAS protocols are not synonymous with clinical pathways because ERAS protocols, unlike clinical pathways, requires auditing and analysis of patient outcomes
- The implementation of ERAS protocols in orthopedics has led to a decrease in length of stay with fewer postoperative complications and reduced cost of care
- Comprehensive preoperative evaluations and interventions are invaluable in improving perioperative outcomes and should be addressed before the day of surgery
- Regional anesthetic techniques are safe with a low rate of neurologic injury and are associated with greater rates of discharge home compared with those receiving general anesthesia.
- ERAS protocols are instrumental in the ambulatory setting due to their emphasis on multimodal analgesia, early mobilization, normothermia, and PONV prophylaxis

ERAS AND ORTHOPEDICS

The early use of a standardized protocol for improving outcomes in orthopedic surgery began in the 1990s at The Hospital for Special Surgery in New York City. Patients there undergoing hip or knee replacement received epidural anesthesia instead of general,

[a] Department of Anesthesiology, Weill Cornell Medicine, 525 East 68th Street, Box 124, New York, NY 10065, USA; [b] Department of Anesthesiology and Pain Medicine, Columbia University Irving Medical Center, 622 West 168th Street, New York, NY 10032, USA; [c] Virginia Commonwealth University, VCU School of Medicine, VCU Department of Anesthesiology, West Hospital, 1200 East Broad Street, 7th Floor, North Wing, Box 980695, Richmond, Virginia 23298, USA
* Corresponding author.
E-mail address: MarissaWeberMD@gmail.com

Clin Sports Med 41 (2022) 345–355
https://doi.org/10.1016/j.csm.2021.11.007
0278-5919/22/© 2021 Elsevier Inc. All rights reserved.

sportsmed.theclinics.com

invasive hemodynamic monitoring, continuous pulse oximetry intraoperatively, and supplemental oxygen in the postoperative period.[1] Through these interventions the observed mortality rate for total knee arthroplasty decreased from 0.44% to 0.07%.[1]

These described clinical care improvements were followed by the development of clinical protocols focused on patient education, multimodal analgesia, and early mobilization after surgery.[2] Institutions like the Mayo Clinic developed a Regional Anesthesia Clinical pathway using opioid-sparing multimodal analgesia and regional anesthetic techniques. Their pathway was shown to provide superior analgesia, fewer postoperative complications, shorter hospital stays, and a reduction of cost.[3] As the volume of orthopedic surgeries have continued to increase, the demand for improved outcomes and higher patient satisfaction will continue to push the development of effective and standardized ERAS protocols.[4]

Despite its earlier advancement in protocolizing pathways to improve patient outcomes, ERAS protocols are still new in orthopedics. Total knee and total hip arthroplasty are the most commonly performed surgeries, and as such, they offer the most data with an officially established protocol published by the ERAS Society in 2019. Recently, aspects of ERAS protocols are being applied to other orthopedic procedures including total shoulder arthroplasty, revisions, and neck of femur fractures; however, the society has not yet developed a formal protocol for these procedures.[5] This article addresses some of the most important aspects of the formal ERAS guidelines for hip and knee arthroplasty, the benefits associated with their implementation, and some important perioperative considerations that are not currently addressed in the guidelines.

HISTORY OF ENHANCED RECOVERY AFTER SURGERY

Enhanced Recovery After Surgery (ERAS) is a multidisciplinary, multimodal, protocolized perioperative clinical care approach designed to improve and expedite the recovery of patients undergoing surgery. The concept of ERAS was originally developed by Dr Henrik Kehlet, a Danish colorectal surgeon, studying perioperative practices to decrease length of stay and improve outcomes after surgery.[6] He proposed that multimodal interventions may lead to a major reduction in the undesirable outcomes from the stress of surgery, accelerated recovery, and a reduction in postoperative morbidity and overall costs.[6,7] In 2001, a group of European academic surgeons, led by Ken Fearon and Olle Ljungqvist, founded an ERAS Study Group.[7] The group aimed to develop a multimodal surgical care pathway based on evidence to improve quality of practice and reduce complications at their respective academic centers. The ERAS Society was officially established in 2010 in Sweden to promote and share ERAS research, improve practice protocols, expand education around perioperative care, and assist with implementation and program auditing.[7]

COMPONENTS OF ERAS AND GOALS

ERAS protocols are comprehensive, multimodal, perioperative care pathways aimed at attenuating the surgical stress response and reducing end-organ dysfunction. The ERAS Society has estimated that there are 20 components of care that influence the stress response and enhance recovery.[8] These elements are grouped according to the timing of the intervention: preoperative, intraoperative, or postoperative.[9] Undertaking such a large endeavor requires a multidisciplinary approach with surgery, anesthesia, nursing, physical therapy, medicine and nutrition all weighing in on implementing protocols.

The preoperative period allows ample opportunities for intervention. The main aspects of ERAS that we focus on include patient education, managing expectations and anxiety, and addressing nutritional strategies including carbohydrate loading and avoiding prolonged fasting. We also address important patient optimization strategies not included in the guidelines but increasingly encountered in clinical care, namely, the management of patients on preoperative opioids and management of patients with opioid use disorder (OUD). Our focus on the intraoperative aspects of ERAS largely addresses the standardization of anesthetic and analgesic regimens using multimodal and regional therapies. Last, we focus on the postoperative interventions that address early mobilization and deep venous thrombosis (DVT) prevention.[9]

WHAT IS ERAS?

It is important to note the distinction between ERAS and other recognized pathways of clinical care. ERAS protocols require compliance with ERAS guidelines and collection and analysis of patient outcomes.[10] Clinical pathways may follow a set of evidenced-based orders and interventions, but they do not require audit and analysis as ERAS protocols do. This difference is critical because unlike clinical pathways, ERAS protocols are used in a standardizing process to facilitate consensus and research within the field.[10]

BENEFITS OF IMPLEMENTING ERAS PROTOCOLS

The vast burden of hospitalization costs lies in postoperative care including physical and occupational therapy, nutrition, and social services.[11] To address this burden, ERAS programs are designed to improve patient outcomes while at the same time limiting cost and decreasing readmission rates after surgery. The concept of ERAS and its increased safety and efficacy in many orthopedic surgeries is lacking, but total joint offers the most data demonstrating a decrease in the length of hospital stay from 4-12 to 1-3 days with no significant increase in all-cause readmission.[12]

PREOPERATIVE PATIENT EDUCATION

Patient education is an important, but unfortunately often overlooked aspect of the perioperative experience. Undergoing surgery is a major life event for most patients. Preoperative education is a useful tool to improve a patient's surgical experience and assist with managing their anxiety and preparing them for the upcoming procedure.[13] Preoperative education should include an explanation of the perioperative process, joint education classes, and an explanation of the type of anesthesia they will receive. Comprehensive analgesia plans should also be discussed to encourage expectation management and assist patients in being active stakeholders in their care.

PERIOPERATIVE ANXIETY REDUCTION

The ERAS guidelines for total knee and hip arthroplasty acknowledge the need for further evidence to demonstrate that preoperative patient education independently reduces the length of hospital stay.[13] Despite this, patient education focusing on anticipated surgical and anesthetic experiences remains a strong recommendation in ERAS guidelines because of the abundance of qualitative evidence demonstrating patient benefit.[13]

Although evidence of a direct association between patient education and a reduction in hospital length of stay remains to be ascertained, studies have demonstrated an independent association between anxiety reduction and preoperative patient education. Preoperative patient education, however, has been independently associated with reduced anxiety in the perioperative period.[13] Beside the psychological benefit this offers patients, there is a profound physical benefit associated with anxiety reduction. Multiple studies have shown a link between anxiety and the development of opiod use disorder (OUD).[14] Persistent opioid use, defined by continued opioid consumption for 90 to 180 days postoperatively, is of great concern because of the associated costs to both the patient and the health care system.[14] Anxiety is also associated with an increased risk of chronic postsurgical pain, a condition defined by persistent pain lasting 2 months after a procedure.[14] Given the significance of developing either of these syndromes on a patient's quality of life after surgery, management of preoperative anxiety through adequate education is critical.

Determining which patients will benefit the most from intervention to reduce anxiety can be challenging. A useful tool to assess patients is the Hospital Anxiety and Depression Scale, which is used to identify patients who may benefit from behavioral interventions like mindfulness-based cognitive therapy or cognitive behavioral therapy before surgery.[14] These behavioral interventions have been a popular treatment for postoperative management of persistent pain; however, recently they have been used to prevent the development of these conditions. A meta-analysis of 4908 patients undergoing orthopedic surgery found that targeted cognitive and behavioral techniques in the preoperative period resulted in improved postoperative pain and perioperative anxiety.[15] The physiologic links between anxiety and postoperative pain are only now being uncovered. A study by Broadbent and colleagues[16] found that increased psychological stress correlated directly to interleukin-1 levels in patients undergoing abdominal surgery. Further studies conducted have shown that a 45-minute relaxation and guided imagery session before and following surgery resulted in improved wound healing.[17] Although there remains much to learn about the mind-body connection in the perioperative period, these interventions that are inexpensive and relatively easy to implement should not be overlooked in preoperative patient education.

PREOPERATIVE MANAGEMENT FOR PATIENTS WITH CHRONIC PAIN

ERAS does not provide specific guidelines for patients with chronic pain on chronic opioid therapy. However, given that an estimated 9% to 35% of the population is on long-term opioid therapy for pain management, it is worth briefly discussing the implications of this trend.[14] Several studies have demonstrated an association between perioperative opioid use and longer hospital stays, greater rates of readmission, and increased postoperative morbidity.[14] In part due to central sensitization and opioid-induced hyperalgesia, patients taking long-term opioids tend to be more sensitive to painful conditions than patients who do not.[18] Even patients on low-dose opioid therapy for osteoarthritic pain before joint arthroplasty were found to have preoperative hyperalgesia and increased risk for postoperative pain.[18] Unsurprisingly, patients using opioids preoperatively are also at higher risk for persistent opioid use.[18]

Until recently, patients with chronic pain were managed primarily with multimodal therapy without any preoperative reduction in their opioid use.[14] A recent study evaluating total joint arthroplasty in long-term opioid users compared those who underwent a 50% reduction in their opioid dose with those who did not. The study found that the prior group had improved functional outcome scores and improved outcomes compared with the group that did not taper before surgery.[14,18] This concept remains a relatively new one that has no place in the formal ERAS guidelines. However, given the size of this population, further research and data about managing long-term opioids before surgery is crucial.

PREOPERATIVE MANAGEMENT OF PATIENTS WITH SUBSTANCE USE DISORDER

The ERAS guidelines do not specifically discuss the management of patients with substance use disorder. However, given the prevalence of the opioid epidemic, it is also worth discussing the management of this unique population here. The most common medications prescribed for patients with OUD include methadone, a μ-opioid agonist with N-methyl-D-aspartate receptor antagonist activity; naltrexone, a μ opioid antagonist; and buprenorphine, a partial μ opioid agonist with high affinity for the μ receptor. Patients on methadone should be continued on their regimen throughout the perioperative period. Although methadone has analgesic properties, additional analgesics will be required in patients receiving surgery who are taking methadone for OUD.[14] Naltrexone, on the other hand, should be discontinued preoperatively in patients who will require opioid analgesics during and after surgery because it will completely block opioid receptors for 72 hours or 4 weeks depending on its formulation.[14]

The guidelines for patients on buprenorphine therapy for OUD are more challenging. Owing to its high affinity for μ receptors, buprenorphine prevents other opioid agonists like dilaudid from binding the μ receptor.[19] Although this pharmacology is ideal in patients with OUD, it is problematic for patients undergoing surgery. In the past, patients have been advised to wean their buprenorphine 3 to 5 days before surgery while taking oral opioid therapy to manage withdrawal. However, for patients with OUD, this puts them at a high risk of relapse.[19] New research suggests that at certain doses of buprenorphine, patients should instead continue their dosages perioperatively with additional buprenorphine or other multimodal therapies used for pain management.[19] These patients are incredibly vulnerable in the perioperative period. It is critical to address goals for pain control and pain management with them and their outpatient providers before surgery to reduce the risk of relapse or inadequate analgesia.[19]

PREOPERATIVE FASTING TIME AND NUTRITION

Preoperative fasting guidelines were developed to reduce the risk of pulmonary aspiration and its associated complications.[20] More recently, hypoglycemia and patient comfort have been recognized as negative consequences of strict fasting guidelines. The current nil per os practice requires waiting 2 hours after ingestion of clear liquids, 6 hours after nonhuman milk and light meals, and 8 hours after heavy meals.[20] Agents used to aid in decreasing gastric volume and/or pH are not currently recommended as part of the ERAS guidelines; however, they may be appropriate in a patient who has risk factors for aspiration.[20]

Recent studies have demonstrated that consumption of a carbohydrate-rich, low-osmolality clear beverages up to 2 hours before surgery can improve perioperative insulin resistance, decrease the risk of postoperative nausea and vomiting, and improve patient satisfaction without adversely affecting gastric emptying and increasing aspiration risk.[21] ERAS protocols have used carbohydrate loading to improve the recovery process with such programs demonstrating shorter hospital length of stays and faster return to function.[22]

INTRAOPERATIVE ANESTHETIC TECHNIQUE

Choosing the optimal anesthetic to minimize surgical duration and complications and modulating the sympathetic response to surgery is a major aspect of the ERAS pathway. Based on the superiority of neuraxial anesthesia over general anesthesia in patients undergoing lower-extremity arthroplasty, ERAS guidelines strongly recommend the use of neuraxial anesthesia for patients undergoing these procedures.[13] These benefits were recognized in 2012 by McDonald and colleagues[23] who used epidural anesthesia techniques in 1081 patients undergoing primary knee arthroplasty with great success.[13] In 2014 Khan and colleagues expanded on this evidence publishing the largest review of enhanced recovery arthroplasty evaluating patients who received spinal anesthesia.[24] Their multiyear retrospective review demonstrated that patients in the enhanced recovery pathway at their institution receiving spinal anesthesia had decreased length of stay (LOS), decreased blood transfusion rates, and decreased incidence of myocardial ischemia within 30 days.[24] These relationships were further demonstrated in Memtsoudis and colleagues's[25] large epidemiologic review of 382,236 patients undergoing primary hip or knee arthroplasty. Their study found that when neuraxial anesthesia was used, 30-day mortality was significantly lower, as was the incidence of a prolonged admission and cost of hospitalization.[25]

As many orthopedic procedures are increasingly performed in an aging population at higher risk for cardiopulmonary complications, we must offer an anesthetic technique that best suits this population. Spinal anesthesia for patients undergoing total knee and total hip arthroplasty is associated with lower rates of transfusion and fewer cardiac events intraoperatively and postoperatively.[26] In the aging population, which is at higher risk for cardiopulmonary complications during and after surgery, the reduction in these risks is profound. Neuraxial techniques have also demonstrated a decreased 90-day mortality with shorter hospital length of stay and no increase in readmission rates.[26] In patients with increased risk for prolonged admission like those with type 2 diabetes, ERAS pathways with spinal anesthetics improved outcomes.[27] A 2015 study demonstrated that type 2 diabetic patients undergoing primary hip and knee arthroplasty under spinal anesthesia were not at increased risk for prolonged hospital admissions.[28] With an increase in chronic diseases, these benefits are crucial in improving both outcomes and cost reduction.

ERAS AND ANALGESIA

From its foundation, the ERAS guidelines have emphasized the importance of multimodal techniques to improve surgical outcomes; this has been realized most notably in the pathway's approach to analgesia. In the past, opioids were used as the primary treatment modality for perioperative pain. However, opioids only target certain receptor pathways and can cause undesirable complications like nausea, constipation, and pruritis. The use of multimodal pain medications instead targets multiple different receptors involved in the pain pathways, all working synergistically together to improve pain relief.

Owing to its safety profile and benefit, preoperative acetaminophen use is strongly recommended in ERAS guidelines.[13] Acetaminophen given preoperatively has been found to both reduce morphine consumption and decrease pain scores in patients undergoing hip and knee arthroplasty.[29] Nonsteroidal anti-inflammatory drugs (NSAIDs) also play an important role in the preoperative period. In 2008, perioperative Celebrex was found to significantly improve postoperative pain scores with decreased opioid consumption and increased range of motion without an increased risk of bleeding.[30] The ERAS guidelines for hip and knee arthroplasty recommend NSAID use perioperatively, but they also recommend that careful patient selection is used when including NSAIDs in an ERAS pathway. A 2016 study by Bjerregaard and colleagues[31] assessed 54 patients who developed a serious renal or urologic complication after undergoing a fast-track hip or knee arthroplasty. Of those 54 patients, 25 had a glomerular filtration rate (GFR) less than 60 before surgery and 16 of those had received a preoperative NSAID.[31]

Gabapentanoids have also been used as part of a multimodal analgesic regimen. However, there have been conflicting data presented regarding their efficacy. One meta-analysis including 7 separate studies published in 2016 assessed gabapentin and pregabalin's effect on postoperative morphine use in patients undergoing total hip arthroplasty.[32] This study found a decrease in morphine use with a statistically significant decrease in nausea.[32] However, a meta-analysis published in 2020 also assessed 7 studies of patients receiving gabapentin for total hip and knee arthroplasty and determined there was no morphine use reduction in the group receiving gabapentin.[33] Given the mixed evidence regarding their use and their associated risk of increased sedation, ERAS does not recommend the standardized use of gabapentanoids for patients undergoing hip or knee arthroplasty.[13]

The popularity of ERAS has grown as the effects of the opioid epidemic were increasingly felt worldwide. This, in addition to the recognition of unpleasant opioid side effects, has led to a desire to minimize the perioperative use of opioids for analgesia. However, opioids remain an important tool in managing perioperative pain especially in managing transition period after a peripheral technique wears off.[13] The ERAS guidelines recognize the benefits of opioids when used in a controlled and appropriate fashion and recommend the use of short-acting, oral opioids instead of extended release opioids to ensure a speedier functional recovery.[13]

ERAS AND PERIPHERAL NERVE BLOCKS

The use of regional techniques both to avoid general anesthesia in patients undergoing joint arthroplasty and to improve postoperative analgesia has continued to gain in popularity. Peripheral nerve blocks (PNBs) use local anesthetics that act via sodium channel blockade to prevent nerve signal propagation along the spinal cord.[34] PNBs can be used in surgery to decrease the anesthetic requirements intraoperatively and improve pain postoperatively. These blocks provide analgesia for up to 24 hours and reduce the number of opioids required by the patient for postoperative pain management.[10] The most commonly performed nerve blocks in joint surgeries include the adductor canal and infiltration between the popliteal artery and the capsule of the posterior knee blocks (I-PACK) for total knee arthroplasty or the interscalene block for total shoulder arthroplasty.

The official ERAS guidelines for PNB after knee arthroplasty do not require the use of PNBs as an essential component of the ERAS pathway[13]; they recognize the superior analgesia provided by a femoral nerve block (FNB) but note concern because of its effect on limiting mobility due to quadriceps weakness. However, PNBs remain a mainstay of therapy for patients undergoing total knee arthroplasty at many institutions. Studies have demonstrated that the adductor canal block (ACB), a variation of the FNB, does not significantly affect quadriceps strength or interfere with ambulation.[35] In addition, studies have demonstrated that the ACB provides equal analgesic benefit to the FNB for patients undergoing total knee arthroplasty.[36] Another new addition, the I-PACK block, has also grown in popularity. Unlike the ACB, which offers motor sparing analgesia for saphenous nerve in the anterior and medial distribution of the joint, the I-PACK block provides motor-sparing analgesia to the posterior joint. The combination of these blocks with periarticular injection (PAI) of local anesthetic has demonstrated superior analgesia for patients undergoing total knee arthroplasty.[37] A recent study assessed those receiving a combination of I-PACK, PAI, and ACB and found that this group had significantly lower pain scores on ambulation on post-op day (POD) 0 to 2 with less opioid consumption throughout their postoperative course.[37]

CONTINUOUS PERIPHERAL NERVE CATHETERS

Although single-shot PNBs have been found to provide excellent analgesia for the first 18 to 24 hours after surgery, placing a peripheral nerve catheter can significantly improve pain control for several days after surgery. Peripheral nerve catheters function by local anesthetic deposition either perineurally or in a muscle plane containing distal branches of nerves. Patients receiving continuous adductor canal catheters for postoperative analgesia after total knee arthroplasty were compared with those receiving single-shot adductor canal and I-PACK blocks. The patients who received catheters had better pain control at rest and with ambulation, consumed less opioids, and demonstrated improved ambulation postoperatively.[38] Although patients with peripheral nerve catheters often remain inpatient for catheter monitoring and local anesthetic infusions, this is not a necessity. With the development of disposable or reuseable, simplified pain pumps, patients are able to be discharged home with peripheral nerve catheters that provide a continuous infusion of local anesthetic for several days postoperatively thus facilitating early postoperative discharge and improving multiple outcomes.

POSTOPERATIVE NAUSEA AND VOMITING

Across all specialties, ERAS recognizes that importance of decreasing postoperative nausea and vomiting (PONV). PONV delays early nutritional intake, causes significant discomfort, and delays discharge.[34] As such, the guidelines recommend screening and multimodal PONV prophylaxis as appropriate.[13] This risk can further be minimized with the use of regional anesthetic techniques including the avoidance of general anesthesia, reduction of opioids, and avoidance of PONV triggering agents. Risk factors for PONV include young age, female sex, nonsmoking, a history of PONV, or a surgery lasting more than 30 minutes.[34]

ANTIMICROBIAL THERAPY

Infection after total joint arthroplasty can be very challenging to manage. Although each institution provides a different antibiotic prophylaxis in the perioperative period, the most recent evidence suggests first- or second-generation cephalosporin therapy dosed within an hour of incision with the addition of vancomycin for patients at increased risk for *Staphylococcus aureus* colonization.[39] Antibiotic-treated cement has received some attention due to the concern for infection after arthroplasty; however, it is not currently recommended in the ERAS guidelines due to a lack of evidence for its use.[13]

NORMOTHERMIA

Anesthesia induces a temperature decrease of 1°C to 2°C in the first hour of surgery followed by a gradual decrease in temperature throughout the surgery.[11] Hypothermia has multiple adverse effects on patient outcomes most notably a worsening of coagulopathy, impairments in wound healing, and an increased risk of infection.[13] Thus, it is imperative to use forced air warming to maintain normothermia both before and during anesthesia to reduce the incidence of hypothermia.

STRATEGIES TO REDUCE BLOOD LOSS

Even with the decreased risk of transmission of infectious disease, blood transfusion is not without risk; it can be associated with coagulopathy, transmission of disease, renal failure, and even death.[13] However, anemia secondary to blood loss also carries an increased risk of infection and mortality.[13] As a result, strategies to reduce intraoperative bleeding during hip and knee arthroplasty are crucial. Tranexamic acid reduces the destruction of fibrin, the protein responsible for blood clot formation; it has been proven to be efficacious in reducing intraoperative blood loss and reducing the need for postoperative transfusion.[40] Tourniquets also reduce blood loss with little risk of nerve injury or ischemic injury as long as appropriate inflation times are followed. As such both receive strong recommendations in the ERAS protocols.[13]

MOBILIZATION AND DVT PROPHYLAXIS

During the perioperative period, patients are also at increased risk for thromboembolic events. Early mobilization and pharmacologic thromboprophylaxis are critical in reducing this risk.[10] Early ambulation is also linked to a shorter length of hospitalization and a lower risk of insulin resistance, muscle atrophy, and pulmonary dysfunction.[13]

CONTINUOUS IMPROVEMENT AND LOOKING FORWARD

The development of ERAS protocols will continue to evolve with the collection and analysis of patient outcomes and further advances in practice. However, the continued success of ERAS depends on compliance with protocols to allow for further consensus and research within the field. Despite its success, the implementation of ERAS protocols remains inconsistent. Even in colorectal surgery, where ERAS was first developed, the compliance with ERAS protocols remains around 60%.[13] The reasons for this are likely varied. However, the benefits offered by these protocols cannot be overlooked. ERAS consistently offers improved patient satisfaction, a decrease in morbidity and mortality, shorter hospital stays, and reduced cost. In the ever-changing health care system with more complex patients and institutional demands, these guidelines are instrumental in delivering the highest standards of patient care.

DISCLOSURE

"The authors have nothing to disclose."

REFERENCES

1. Sharrock NE, Cazan MG, Hargett MJ, et al. Changes in mortality after total hip and knee arthroplasty over a ten-year period. Anesth Analg 1995;80:242–8.
2. Duggal S, Flics S, Cornell CN. Introduction of clinical path- ways in orthopedic surgical care: the experience of the hospital for special surgery. In: MacKenzie CR, Cornell CN, Memtsoudis SG, editors. Perioperative care of the orthopedic patient. New York: Springer; 2014. p. 365–71.
3. Duncan CM, Moeschler SM, Horlocker TT, et al. A self-paired comparison of perioperative out- comes before and after implementation of a clinical path- way in patients undergoing total knee arthroplasty. Reg Anesth Pain Med 2013;38: 533–8.
4. Kaye AD, Urman RD, Cornett EM, et al. Enhanced recovery pathways in orthopedic surgery. J Anaesthesiol Clin Pharmacol 2019;35(Suppl 1):S35–9.
5. C. Ronald MacKenzia, Charles N. Cornell, Stavros G. Memtsoudis. Perioperative care of the orthopedic patient (Kindle Locations 7035-7036). Springer International Publishing. Kindle Edition. 2014.
6. Kehlet H. Multimodal approach to control postoperative pathophysiology and rehabilitation. Br J Anaesth 1997;78(5):606–17.

7. Kehlet H, Mogensen T. Hospital stay of 2 days after open sigmoidectomy with a multimodal rehabilitation program. Br J Surg 1999;86(2):227–30.

8. Tanious MK, Ljungqvist O, Urman RD. Enhanced recovery after surgery: history, evolution, guidelines, and future directions. Int Anesthesiol Clin 2017;55(4):1–11.

9. Varadhan KK, Lobo DN, Ljungqvist O. Enhanced recovery after surgery: the future of improving surgical care. Crit Care Clin 2010;26(3):527–47.

10. Soffin EM, YaDeau JT. Enhanced recovery after surgery for primary hip and knee arthroplasty: a review of the evidence. Br J Anaesth 2016;117(suppl 3). https://doi.org/10.1093/bja/aew362. iii62-iii72.

11. Malviya A, Martin K, Harper I, et al. Enhanced recovery program for hip and knee replacement reduces death rate. Acta Orthop 2011;82(5):577–81.

12. Zhu S, Qian W, Jiang C, et al. Enhanced recovery after surgery for hip and knee arthroplasty: a systematic review and meta-analysis. Postgrad Med J 2017;93(1106):736–42.

13. Wainwright TW, Gill M, McDonald DA, et al. Consensus statement for perioperative care in total hip replacement and total knee replacement surgery: Enhanced Recovery After Surgery (ERAS) Society recommendations. Acta Orthopaedica 2019;91(1):3–19.

14. Doan LV, Blitz J. Preoperative assessment and management of patients with pain and anxiety disorders. Curr Anesthesiology Rep 2020;10(1):28–34.

15. Szeverenyi C, Kekecs Z, Johnson A, et al. The use of adjunct psychosocial interventions can decrease postoperative pain and improve the quality of clinical care in orthopedic surgery: a systematic review and meta-analysis of randomized controlled trials. J Pain 2018 Nov;19(11):1231–52.

16. Broadbent E, Petrie KJ, Alley PG, et al. Psychological stress impairs early wound repair following surgery. Psychosom Med 2003;65(5):865–9.

17. Broadbent E, Kahokehr A, Booth RJ, et al. A brief relaxation intervention reduces stress and improves surgical wound healing response: A randomized trial. Brain Behav Immun 2012;26(2):212–7.

18. Miclescu A. Chronic pain patient and anaesthesia. Rom J Anaesth Intensive Care 2019;26(1):59–66.

19. Ward EN, Quaye AN, Wilens TE. Opioid use disorders: perioperative management of a special population. Anesth Analg 2018;127(2):539–47.

20. Abe K, Adelhoj B, Andersson H, et al. Practice guidelines for preoperative fasting and the use of pharmacologic agents to reduce the risk of pulmonary aspiration: application to healthy patients undergoing elective procedures. Anesthesiology 2017;126(3):376–93.

21. Melnyk M, Casey RG, Black P, et al. Enhanced recovery after surgery (ERAS) protocols: Time to change practice? Can Urol Assoc J 2011;5(5):342–8.

22. Kratzing C. Pre-operative nutrition and carbohydrate loading. Proc Nutr Soc 2011;70(3):311–5.

23. McDonald DA, Siegmeth R, Deakin AH, et al. An enhanced recovery program for primary total knee arthroplasty in the United Kingdom: follow up at one year. Knee 2012;19(5):525–9.

24. Khan SK, Malviya A, Muller SD, et al. Reduced short-term complications and mortality following enhanced recovery primary hip and knee arthroplasty: results from 6,000 consecutive procedures. Acta Orthop 2014;85(1):26–31.

25. Memtsoudis SG, Sun X, Chiu YL, et al. Perioperative comparative effectiveness of anesthetic technique in orthopedic patients. Anesthesiology 2013;118(5):1046–58.

26. Hutton M, Brull R, Macfarlane AJR. Regional anaesthesia and outcomes. BJA Educ 2018;18(2):52–6.
27. Beverly A, Kaye AD, Ljungqvist O, et al. Essential elements of multimodal analgesia in enhanced recovery after surgery (ERAS) Guidelines. Anesthesiol Clin 2017;35(2):115–43.
28. Jorgensen CC, Madsbad S, Kehlet H. Lundbeck Foundation Centre for Fast-track Hip and Knee Replacement Collaborative Group. Postoperative morbidity and mortality in type-2 diabetics after fast-track primary hip and knee arthroplasty. Anesth Analg 2015;120:230–8.
29. Apfel C, Turan A, Souza K, et al. Intravenous acetaminophen reduces postoperative nausea and vomiting: a systematic review and meta-analysis. Pain 2013; 154(5):677–89.
30. Huang YM, Wang CM, Wang CT, et al. Peri- operative celecoxib administration for pain management after total knee arthroplasty: a randomized, controlled study. BMC Musculoskelet Disord 2008;9:77. https://doi.org/10.1186/1471-2474-9-77.
31. Bjerregaard LS, Jorgensen CC, Kehlet H, et al. Serious renal and urological complications in fast-track primary total hip and knee arthroplasty; a detailed observational cohort study. Minerva Anestesiol 2016;2:179–88.
32. Mao Y, Wu L, Ding W. The efficacy of preoperative administration of gabapentin/pregabalin in improving pain after total hip arthroplasty: a meta-analysis. BMC Musculoskelet Disord 2016;17(1):373.
33. Kang J, Zhao Z, Lv J, et al. The efficacy of perioperative gabapentin for the treatment of postoperative pain following total knee and hip arthroplasty: a meta-analysis. J Orthop Surg Res 2020;15:332. https://doi.org/10.1186/s13018-020-01849-6.
34. Butterworth JF, Wasnick JD, Mackey DC. In: Malley J, editor. Clinical anesthesiology. 6th edition. C. Naglieri. 6th edition. McGraw-Hill Education; 2018.
35. Jaeger P, Nielsen ZJ, Henningsen MH, et al. Adductor canal block versus femoral nerve block and quadriceps strength: a randomized, double-blind, placebo-controlled, crossover study in healthy volunteers. Anesthesiology 2013;118(2): 409–15.
36. Kuang MJ, Xu LY, Ma JX, et al. Adductor canal block versus continuous femoral nerve block in primary total knee arthroplasty: A meta-analysis. Int J Surg 2016; 31:17–24.
37. Kim DH, Beathe JC, Lin Y, et al. Addition of infiltration between the popliteal artery and the capsule of the posterior knee and adductor canal block to periarticular injection enhances postoperative pain control in total knee arthroplasty: a randomized controlled trial. Anesth Analg 2019;129(2):526–35.
38. Tak R, Gurava Reddy AV, Jhakotia K, et al. Continuous adductor canal block is superior to adductor canal block alone or adductor canal block combined with IPACK block (interspace between the popliteal artery and the posterior capsule of knee) in postoperative analgesia and ambulation following total knee arthroplasty: randomized control trial. Musculoskelet Surg 2020. https://doi.org/10.1007/s12306-020-00682-8.
39. Goswami Karan, Kimberley L. Stevenson, javad parvizi, intraoperative and postoperative infection prevention. J Arthroplasty 2020;35(3). https://doi.org/10.1016/j.arth.2019.10.061. S2-S8, ISSN 0883-5403.
40. Fillingham YA, Ramkumar DB, Jevsevar DS, et al. The efficacy of tranexamic acid in total knee arthroplasty: a network meta-analysis. J Arthroplasty 2018;33(10): 3090–8.e1.

Moving?

Make sure your subscription moves with you!

To notify us of your new address, find your **Clinics Account Number** (located on your mailing label above your name), and contact customer service at:

Email: journalscustomerservice-usa@elsevier.com

800-654-2452 (subscribers in the U.S. & Canada)
314-447-8871 (subscribers outside of the U.S. & Canada)

Fax number: 314-447-8029

Elsevier Health Sciences Division
Subscription Customer Service
3251 Riverport Lane
Maryland Heights, MO 63043

*To ensure uninterrupted delivery of your subscription, please notify us at least 4 weeks in advance of move.